Meanwood Park Hospital
A Home for the 'Misunderstood'

Ross Farrally

Printing by *Book Printing* UK

Copyright © 2020 Ross Farrally

All rights reserved. No part of this publication may be reproduced, distributed, or transmitted in any form or by any means, including photocopying, recording, or other electronic or mechanical methods, without the prior written permission of the publisher, except in the case of brief quotations in critical reviews and certain other non-commercial uses permitted by copyright law. For permission requests, write to the publisher at the address below.

Publisher: Ross Publishing

Publication date: 08.12.2020

ISBN: 978-1-80049-188-5 (Paperback)

Front cover image by Ross Farrally
Book design by Ross Farrally

First printing edition 2021

Printing: Book Printing UK

rosspublishing.net
www.facebook.com/rosspublishing
ross@rosspublishing.net

DISCLAIMER

The purpose of this book is to provide you, the reader, an insight into Meanwood Park Hospital using interviews with former staff and volunteers. Interviews were carried out in a variety of ways and all interviewees were supplied with the final copy in which they gave their permission for publication. To ensure the protection of identities of all those involved, names and characteristics have been altered unless agreed with the interviewee.

This is also not a case study of the institution; this book is merely a collection of interviews with the addition of a brief history of the hospital and a short history of learning disabilities. Due to the history of this disability, please be aware that old terminology has been used in parts of this book. Today, this former terminology is severely outdated, offensive, and degrading.

With my initial knowledge on Meanwood Park Hospital being thin, I spent a lengthy period researching the hospital using a variety of sources. These came in the form of medical journals, parliament meeting notes, historical newspaper articles, original documents, websites and the knowledge of the interviewees. Websites that have been used have been referenced at the close of this book.

Regardless of the time spent looking into the history of the former hospital, I have tried with the utmost commitment to ensure that everything written in this book is factual and accurate to the best of my knowledge. I would like to apologise beforehand if anything you read may not be entirely correct but please be aware, I have gone to great lengths to prevent this.

Bad language is also found in a select few interviews.

To finalize, the views and opinions expressed in this book are those of the author and not necessarily reflect the official policy or position or any other agency, organization, employer, or company.

***

ACKNOWLEDGEMENTS

Books comprised of interviews are solely built by the individuals who come forward to tell their stories and I would like to express my deepest appreciation to those who reached out to me. It is your extensive memories that allow institutions such as Meanwood Park Hospital to live on, providing future generations with an insight into these historic times.

Meanwood Park Hospital would have remained a mystery to myself if it weren't for my sister Kimberley. She introduced me to housing estate which sits on the former grounds and provided me with my first visit to the mansion. Her support and input in these books will be forever appreciated.

An immeasurable level of appreciation goes to David Foster who supplied me with invaluable memorabilia of Meanwood Park Hospital. David provided me with original documents, photographs, booklets and was kind enough to produce a detailed map of the hospital. I will forever be grateful for David's input in this book.

Finally, I would like to recognize my family and friends. Their ongoing support has helped make these books transition from ideas to reality.

***

CONTENTS

Introduction	8
Meanwood Park Hospital	10
Learning Disabilities	20
1940s *to* 1960s	
Joan McGrail	31
Gordon Greaves	33
Laurel Macy	35
Robert Spinks	40
1970s	
David Foster	43
Amelia Brown	62
Grace Jones	67
Sarah Read	74
1980s *to* 1990s	
Margaret Hartley	88
Chris Gordon	84
Victoria Wolfe	103
Hannah Heaton	108
George Walker	122
Adam Heaton	135
Jenna Craig	139
Terry Craig	146
Rosie Hope	152
Leanne Firth	155
Summary	160
Libby Hays	162
More from the Author	170
An Insight into 'Insanity'	171
References	175

INTRODUCTION

High Royds Hospital: An Insight into 'Insanity' was my first venture into the world of literature. I was thankful that my knowledge of the institution was praised by those who read it.

Meanwood Park Hospital: A Home for the 'Misunderstood' was formed from the public's desire to know more about the former hospital. It was a mystery to me, much like it still may be to those who live in the estate and the surrounding areas. I was lucky enough to have more than twelve-years knowledge of High Royds Hospital however, my understanding of Meanwood Park Hospital has only been present for seven-years, thereabouts.

Unless you had personal connections to Meanwood Park Hospital, you are more than likely unaware, to an extent, of the type of care that it offered to its residents. The thought of segregating those with learning disabilities, by today's standards, is unnecessary and creates that divide of 'other'. Select philosophies present during the early 20th century promoted the incarceration of these individuals, one of these ideologies was promoted by the Eugenics Society. They believed that the social ills associated to these individuals would spread amongst offspring which would gradually wear away at "society's physical, intellectual and moral core, resulting in its eventual collapse."[1] This claim inevitably led to the segregation of these individuals from the rest of society.

I am an example that you do not need to have an English degree or university degree in journalism to produce a book on a subject you have enthusiasm for. Local history depends on us, it is reliant on those with interests to keep stories of the past, stories of places like Meanwood Park Hospital, alive.

Meanwood Park Hospital: A Home for the 'Misunderstood' provides an insight into a time where those with learning disabilities were not treated as equal members of society.

***

MEANWOOD PARK HOSPITAL

Meanwood Park Hospital has an extensive history and due to that, I decided to give only a brief outline of the most significant events that I thought were beneficial for this book.

Meanwood Hall, the mansion that remains upright today, was constructed circa-1762 for Thomas Denison. In 1762, Mr Denison purchased a dwelling house plus an additional thirteen acres at Meanwood which, at the time, was known as Hawcaster Rigg in Chapel Allerton. It is here that Thomas built Meanwood Hall.

After his death in 1796, his wife Elizabeth was handed the estate which she later vacated, advertising the Hall in the Leeds Intelligencer, which was one of the first regional newspapers in Great Britain, describing the property as follows:

"Four spacious rooms on the ground floor, with very good bedrooms over, kitchen, pantries, servants' hall, coach house, stabling for ten good horses and about twenty acres of land."[3]

After Elizabeth's death, it was then passed down to her son, Robert Denison, who went on to purchase neighbouring cottages which he, in turn, demolished as he wasn't content on them being so close to his mansion.

In the years that followed, the estate was occupied by various tenants including Thomas Turton, the Countess of Aberdeen, Sir John Beckett, who owned two adjacent cottages and Joseph Lees.

In 1814, Joseph Lees was the inhabitant of the Hall and it was in this period that he organised the North Wing extension.

Ten years later, Christopher Beckett, the son of former tenant, Sir John Beckett, purchased the property from Robert Denison, putting an end to over sixty years of Denison Family ownership.

During the mid-1800s, a lodge, which took on the appearance of a typical Victorian home, was constructed at the foot of the main drive. It is believed that this was erected for either Thomas himself, or his two sisters Mary and Elizabeth. The lodge remains in use today as a standard residence.

Developments continued and in 1834, local architect, John Clarke, who designed the mansion in Roundhay Park, made further adjustments to Meanwood Hall.

The Hall remained in the Beckett Family for some time, with Thomas' sisters taking control of the estate after his death in 1847. It remained in the hands of the Beckett's until Elizabeth's passing in 1864 which led to other tenants taking temporary residence until 1872 where the Hall stood unoccupied for three years.

The last known resident of the mansion was R.W Bower, a colliery owner in Allerton. His company, T. & R. W. Bower Ltd, owned four mines in Leeds: Albert, Fleatingley Beck, primrose Hill and Victoria.

In 1919, the Leeds Corporation rented Meanwood Park to provide a colony for the mentally handicapped, which officially opened as the Meanwood Park Colony on the 3rd June 1920 by Sir William Byrne. Despite being formally opened in 1920, the first patient, who went on to be a fixture for over sixty-years, was admitted on the 25th August 1919.

Between 1913 and 1921, Sir William Byrne served as the Chairman of the Board of Control for Lunacy and Mental Deficiency. The body was formed from the creation of the Mental Deficiency Act 1913 with responsibility falling on their shoulders to oversee the treatment of the mentally ill in England and Wales.

When the doors to the colony opened, it originally housed a total of 103 patients. 35 males and 52 females occupied the mansion while the remaining 16 patients were housed in a nearby block. Maps dated 1919 show that the nearest block was located roughly 270-feet north-east of the hall.

Just two-years later, The Meanwood Park estate and its surrounding land were purchased from Sir Hickman Beckett Bacon, grandson of Sir Thomas Beckett, for £14,000.

Sir Hickman Beckett Bacon was a founding member of the Lincolnshire Automobile Club and became president in 1902, a position in which he held until his death in 1945. He was one of the first individuals in Gainsborough to own a car, a Panhard Levassor.

During the 1920s, Samuel Wormald became the notorious Executive Officer of Meanwood Park Colony. His name is etched into the history of the hospital due to his views and actions in relation to those suffering with disabilities. He was known to remove more than 2,000 people from society because he believed that "...by being allowed to repeat their type [have children], the feebleminded are increasing the ranks of the degenerate and wastrel classes with disastrous consequences to the entire community".[4] Samuel deemed individuals as unfit for absurd reasons such as being deaf, blind and dumb – anyone considered to be mentally deficient or imperfect. These people were then plucked from society and confined to the colony. His behaviours led him to being labelled as the ratcatcher.

Prior to his contribution to Meanwood Park Colony, Samuel Wormald was involved in the Eugenics Society. This group "sought to increase public understanding of heredity and to influence parenthood in Britain, with the aim of biological improvement of the nation and mitigation of the burdens deemed to be imposed on society by the genetically 'unfit'."[5] As previously mentioned in the introduction, the Eugenics believed that these defectives would cause a societal collapse if they were allowed to produce offspring. Samuel used his beliefs coupled with his level of authority at the hospital to remove these individuals from the community.

In 1931, a bill was drafted and presented to Parliament by Major A G Church, the MP for Wandsworth. It called for the compulsory sterilisation of mental defectives which ultimately failed, as did successive attempts. It is important to note that a similar programme, named Aktion T4, was carried out in Nazi extermination camps during the Second World War. Adolf Hitler put pen to paper on a euthanasia note and "certain German physicians were authorised to select patients 'deemed incurably sick, after most critical medical examination' and then administer to them a 'mercy death'."[6]

Meanwood Park Colony continued to develop and underwent further expansion in 1923.

By 1928, Meanwood Park Colony required further developments which led to a limited competition being held. The plans of Messrs J. M. Sheppard & Partners, who were architects of London, were selected which would lead to a hospital suitable for 900 patients. Moving forward, the patients were then able to be segregated into male, female, and children. This expansion, along with many others around the country, adopted the use of cottages to house patients, thus removing the feeling of being in a hospital. This style was implemented to create a more suitable living environment as the perception at the time was that these people would remain here for the rest of their lives. The idea that these individuals would remain permanent fixtures of these hospitals triggered the change that they would become known as residents rather than patients.

Prior to their successful plans for Meanwood Park Colony, the architects were also responsible for the design of Cell Barnes Hospital in Tyttenhanger, St Albans. This was another institute for those with mental deficiencies with the layout being similar to that of Meanwood's.

Despite the plans being given the green light in 1928, it wasn't until the 3rd October 1932 that the first segment of this extension was opened by Councillor Arthur Hawkyard, MD, LLS, JP, and Chairman of the Mental Health Committee. This created an additional accommodation for 328 residents, bringing the total number to 433.

Two years after the first extension was completed, Dr Z. P. Fernandez approved the final part of the scheme on the 20th November 1934. The latest development included "seven additional villas, a hospital villa, a villa for the most dependent cases, a recreation hall for 600, a nurses' residence of three storeys with 70 bedrooms, six staff houses, central kitchen, stores, workshops, and a house for the Superintendent."[7] These final extensions provided for an additional 410 patients thus, bringing the total potential capacity to 841.

On the 2nd June 1938, the Victorian dwelling that stood on the corner of Spen Lane, Kirkstall, opened its doors to become the annexe of Meanwood Park Hospital. This residence was known as Crooked Acres and was believed to have been constructed circa-1871 by John Octavius Butler. In the beginning, it was a women's only annexe, with many of the residents leaving the confines of the home to carry out local domestic work. In the years that followed, male patients were integrated, and Crooked Acres became a mixed-sex lodge. The building took on the appearance of a large mid-Victorian, gothic-style villa, complete with bay windows and a conservatory to the south-west. Leading off the conservatory was a set of stone steps that lead down to a grass terrace. Once through the main entrance, residents were met with a small walkway which progressed into the stairway. One noticeable feature to mention was the Italianate, gothic-style marble fireplace that occupied one of the north-west rooms. Today, the lodge, known as Kirkside House, continues its use as a residential home, caring for adults with complex needs and learning disabilities.

In 1939, the hospital appointed Dr Alexander H. Wilson as the first Superintendent. At the time, he was one of the few doctors that specialised in the care of the mentally handicapped and became the main driving force behind the expansion of the hospital's many services, including Crooked Acres.

Come September, with the commencement of World War II, the hospital shifted gears and became an emergency hospital, caring for both British and German troops as well as the local civilians. To meet the demands at the time, an operating theatre was established and remained in use once the war ended, being refurbished into a dental surgery. The residents, prior to this transformation, were crowded into certain villas or moved elsewhere.

Seven years after its approval, the final extensions to the hospital were opened on the 23rd June 1941 by Mary, Princess Royal and Countess of Harewood. Much like the architects' plans for Cell Barnes Hospital, it was now an institution embracing the use of individual villas rather than one large building.

With the rise of the Industrial Revolution, many psychiatric hospitals around the country were introducing Industrial Therapy so their daily regime. Meanwood Park Hospital was no different, with the department undergoing an extension in the 1960s. The aim of Industrial Therapy was to allow the individuals to use the skills that they had required prior to their admittance, to occupy themselves for the benefit of the hospital and as an aid in their treatment.

In 1964, former Superintendent, Dr Alexander H. Wilson, who retired in 1961, opened a new single storey villa for forty mentally and physically handicapped children.

The amount of beds at the hospital peaked at 841 during the 1960s but this subsequently began to fall shortly after.

The emphasis on developing patient care continued with evening classes being provided for in-patients by the Leeds Education Authority.

I was truly fortunate to stumble across Sketches from the history of psychiatry, which was a short piece published by Douglas A. Spencer, a former Consultant Psychiatrist and Senior Clinical Lecturer in 1989. He was kind enough to write a small section on the League of Friends.

"One of the most significant developments in the life-story of Meanwood Park Hospital was the founding of the League of Friends in December 1965. This enabled citizens from the community to bring their time and talents to benefit the hospital. Known as 'The Friends', the league has remembered patients on their birthdays and at Christmas, regularly donated money to the villas, and provided numerous amenities. In addition, the Friends have raised well over £100,000 for eight major projects: the building of the Visitors' Tea-room, twice extended; the Adult Activities Centre; the Leisure and Recreation Department; and three minibuses. For 20 years an annual garden party in the grounds, opened by a celebrity, attracted hundreds of visitors and raised thousands of pounds."[8]

Towards the end of the 1960s, the hospital continued to improve its services by the way of converting the original infirmary block. The renovations paved the way for "an admission, assessment and short-stay unit, with a psychology department, pharmacy, X-ray room, laboratory, consulting rooms and dental suite."[9] The medical staff became further diverse with the team now containing "three consultant psychiatrists, a senior registrar training in mental handicap, a registrar and six clinical assistants."[10] Further changes were implemented in regard to patient comforts, with the addition of an on-site clothing store, shop, and hairdressing salon.

In 1971, Meanwood Park Hospital requested a grant under the Urban Programme by the Leeds City Council for a play centre to be built for a total cost of £156. This was closely followed by a new adult activity centre which was constructed in 1976.

On the back of the evening classes that were implemented in 1965, a pilot day-time Continuing Adult Education scheme, financed by Leeds Education Authority, was inaugurated in 1978.

With psychiatric hospitals around the county beginning to transition into community-based care, it wasn't long until colonies such as Meanwood Park Hospital also felt that pressure to follow suit. In the 1980s, a new special school was constructed beside the hospital and one of the on-site villas was converted into four individual flatlets. Other villas were transformed to create living spaces for eight or ten residents, with the focus turning to rehabilitation. With the hospital moving in a new direction, a Resettlement Officer was appointed with the aim to move suitable in-patients out of the hospital and into more appropriate settings such as community houses or projects run by the local housing association.

By the mid-1980s, the hospital began selling sections of the land, with three villas and the recreation hall falling victim to closure. With the number of in-patients continuing to fall, thus leading to more empty homes, the recreation hall was quickly reintroduced with one of the remaining villas being transformed.

Despite the phased closure of the hospital, in 1989 Meanwood Park Hospital was the biggest hospital for mental handicap in the Yorkshire Health Region, with the number of beds at 340. It is hard to compare these figures with other hospitals due to how they presented their numbers. Some offered information based on resident numbers while others offered beds available. For example, if Meanwood Park Hospital had 100 beds available, it doesn't mean that all of those were filled which makes it difficult to compare that to a hospital who measured via resident numbers. You could argue that the reason why Meanwood Park Hospital was the largest mental handicap hospital in the Yorkshire Region in 1989 was due to that many other colonies closed in previous years such as

Claypenny Colony in 1993, Oulton Hall in 1972 and Stansfield View in 1993.

In May 1997, Meanwood Park Hospital ceased its services, ending approximately seventy-seven years of inpatient healthcare.

***

LEARNING DISABILITIES

"The aim of these early asylums was to train and educate people with learning disabilities."[11]

Before I continue with this piece, I have to repeat the fact that it contains phrases that are no longer used in today's world. It was essential to include these labels as it highlights the general attitude towards the disability in that given time period.

Much like the history of Meanwood Park Hospital, learning disabilities can be traced back to when man first existed and due to that, I will only be covering the periods that I believe are most beneficial.

Some of the first attempts at forming specialist institutions for those with learning disabilities, or as it was referred to then, cretinism, began in 1842 in Switzerland and in Leipzig in 1846.

One significant doctor to reference in this time period was Dr Guggenbuhl who began to study cretinism in 1839. It would be three years later when he opened his school for cretins, located on the Abendburg which is one of the secondary elevations on the Bernese Alps in Western Switzerland. He was "determined to devote his life and energies to the redemption of these lost outcasts of humanity."[12] Dr Guggenbuhl was one of many who believed that cretinism could be cured at high elevations.

This theory dated back three and a quarter centuries via the way of Horace Bénédict de Saussure who exclaimed that "cretinism is rarely, if ever, found higher than an altitude of 3000 feet above the sea."[13]

Horace Bénédict de Saussure recorded his interaction with cretinism in his publication, *Voyages dans les Alpes*. "I asked the first person I met what the name of the village was, and when he did not reply I asked a second, and then a third; but a dismal silence, or a few inarticulate noises were the only response I received. The stupid amazement with which they looked at me, their enormous goitres, their fat, parted lips, their heavy, drooping eyelids, their hanging jaws, their doltish expressions, were quite terrifying. It was as if an evil spirit had transformed every inhabitant into a dumb animal, leaving only the human form to show that they had once been men. I left with an impression of fear and sadness which will never be erased from my memory."[14]

Another doctor by the name of Dr Fodéré assumed that "the removal to a keen, dry mountain air is the main condition for successful treatment."[15]

Through the writings of Dr A. Reed, Dr Twinning and Dr J Conolly, the first English institution was introduced in Bath, being nothing more than a small project contained in the Magdalen Hospital. Prior to the scheme embedding its roots, the hospital was in fact a charitable organization for the rehabilitation of fallen women.

It was Dr J Conolly's involvement at Middlesex County Asylum that ultimately led him to Bath. After being inspired by the work of Seguin in Paris, he conducted his own experiment at the asylum which led him to the conclusion that a separate institution was needed, and this resulted in the creation of Park House Asylum in London.

Park House was purchased in 1848 and became known as The Asylum for Idiots. The building rapidly became unfit for use and a new purpose-built facility was commissioned. Prince Albert, who took a special interest in the institution from the beginning, laid the foundation stone in June 1853 and opened the asylum two years later in June 1855. Seventy-one years later, the hospital would be retitled as The Royal Earlswood Institution for Mental Defectives with the aim to train and educate people with learning disabilities. Due to the conversion into community-based care, the hospital went into decline and closed in 1997.

It was towards the end of the 19th century when the eugenics society came to fruition but as I have already briefly covered this, I will only provide you with the following quote.

"The dangers lie in the fact that these degenerates' mate with healthy members of the community and thereby constantly drag fresh blood into the vortex of disease and lower the general vigour of the nation." (Tredgold, 1909)

With the introduction of The Mental Deficiency Act 1913, individuals with learning disabilities could be involuntarily admitted to the local asylum, many never returning to their families. This was because the Act categorised these people, alongside those with mental health issues, as idiots, imbeciles, feeble-minded or moral defectives. Prolonged institutional care and extreme childhood hardship were two of the many reasons that individuals could be diagnosed with mental deficiency.

The idea that those diagnosed with learning disabilities should be living in segregated communities continued into the 1940s with the introduction of Camphill Communities. This movement was global and involved building devoted societies "where everyone can find purpose and belonging."[16] It would be in Aberdeen, Scotland where the first community was founded, led by Dr Karl König, an Australian paediatrician, and his group of refugees. Prior to his involvement in Scotland, Dr Karl König undertook a paediatrician role at the Rudolf Steiner-inspired Schloß Pilgrimshain institute in Strzegom. After fleeing Vienna due to Hitler's invasion of Austria, he relocated to Aberdeen where, with the help of his group, recommenced his work. It was from his time in Vienna where Dr Karl König and his team found their purpose living and working with children with learning disabilities. It is important to note that during the 1940s, people with learning disabilities were omitted from education and many other dimensions of society. König's view at the time was that "every human being possessed a healthy inner personality that was independent of their physical characteristics, including characteristics marking developmental or mental disability, and the role of the school was to recognize, nurture and educate this essential self." (Marga Hogenboom, 2001) Some of these small populations had their own organic gardens, workshops and bakeries that sold products to the surrounding areas.

Today, there are three of these communities in the Yorkshire region; Pennine Community in West Yorkshire and both Botton Village and the Croft Community in North Yorkshire. The NHS website for Pennine

Camphill Community, also known as Camphill Wakefield, describes the community as follows.

"Pennine Community supports a further education college for students who have learning disabilities. The college supports both residential and day students. Term time accommodation and personal care is available for up to for up to 29 students. The college provides a therapeutic environment and experiential learning opportunities within a craft centre and outdoor learning opportunities."[17]

After the Second World War, Judy Fryd, a mother of a child with learning disabilities, became a revolutionary campaigner for children with learning disabilities and founder of The National Association of Parents of Backwards Children, now known as Mencap. The association was established after her child, Felicity, was rejected from school due to her troublesome behaviour, described then as juvenile schizophrenia. Another school deemed that her child was not suitable which resulted in her immediate removal. It was the lack of support and absence of understanding from professionals and society that became the driving force behind Judy's pioneering work. In 1946, the Nursery World magazine published an article asking if there were any other parents struggling to manage a learning-disabled child at home. Judy was quick to respond, suggesting other affected parents should come together in an effort to obtain some kind of acknowledgement and support for their difficulties and within the month, over one-thousand parents came forward. Through her perseverance, Judy transformed the public's perception of learning disabilities and led a movement which resulted in the introduction of the 1971 Education

(Handicapped Children) Act which overturned the initial assumption that children with learning disabilities were uneducable.

With the formation of the NHS in 1948, institutions around the country were now under the control of the National Health Service and were to be referred to as hospitals.

At the beginning of the 1950s, it was believed that around 55,000 people with learning disabilities were living in hospitals in England and Wales with further research concluding that many of these residents had the skills to live out in the community and undertake paid work.

Research into the institutional care model continued and in 1958, Professor Jack Tizard, a psychologist who "worked at the boundaries of psychology, medicine, education and social sciences"[18] conducted an experiment at the Maudsley Psychiatric Hospital which he entitled the *Brooklands Experiment*. His work revealed that children who lived in small houses in the community developed better than those who lived in hospitals. These results helped with the shift towards deinstitutionalisation and the creation of smaller communities.

The introduction of the Mental Health Act of 1959 called for a more community-based approach, but the numbers of admittances continued to rise which led to more hospitals being constructed to meet the demand. Despite these new institutions being built, conditions continued to reflect that of its predecessors and in March 1969, the Ely Report was presented to Parliament which exposed dreadful treatment of the residents at Ely Hospital.

The hospital served many purposes through its years of service but with the introduction of the NHS, it was designated as a Mental Deficiency Institution and Mental Hospital. The conditions of the hospital were brought into the public eye through the News of the World who obtained its story from a nursing assistant of the hospital. The public outrage that followed led to the founding of a committee who would go on to make a full investigation into the allegations. The gentleman to chair this committee was Geoffrey Howe. It is important to reference Geoffrey as he made the initial strives towards ensuring investigations were made into all of the institutions that cared for people with learning disabilities.

"It was Howe who insisted the inquiry should go far beyond the events at Ely itself, to look at the whole system and the way in which people with learning difficulties – "mental handicap", as it was known at the time – were treated".[19]

I have taken the opportunity to include some extracts from this report which can be seen below.

"XY had been employed as a Nursing Assistant at Ely from 26th September 1966, until 24th September 1967. The full text of his original statement is set out in the Appendix to this Report. The allegations made, which all referred to the male wards at Ely, fell under the following general headings:

- Cruel ill-treatment of four particular patients by six named members of the staff.
- Generally inhumane and threatening behaviour towards patients by one of the staff members already referred to.
- Pilfering of food, clothing and other items belonging to the hospital or the patients.

- Indifference on the part of the Chief Male Nurse to complaints that were made to him.
- Lack of care by the Physician Superintendent and one other member of the medical staff."[20]

The final transcript of evidence amounted to more than one-thousand pages.

The Ely Hospital report is regarded as significant in the advancement of services for these patients. It led to the 1971 white paper *Better Services for the Mentally Handicapped* and the first inspections of such services.

To summarise the above white paper, its focus was to move away from inpatient institutions and increase the provision of local and community care. It is also important to note that the white paper did recognise that in some cases, a hospital setting would be more appropriate. Those who were suitable to live in the community were to be placed in more homely settings such as group-living homes, children's homes and homes for the elderly.

The Jay Report (1979) expanded on the aim of social acceptance by outlining that the lives of people with learning disabilities should be normal and that they should be welcomed into their communities. This was based on the idea of "Normalisation" that had been supported in Denmark since the late 1950s.

"The concept came in form as the piece of Danish legislation introduced by Niels Erik Bank-Mikkelsen called the 1959 Mental Retardation Act, its political aims were to fundamentally change perspectives towards those with intellectual difficulties, hopefully resulting in the group becoming 'normalised' and attaining the same community-based rights as those without disabilities, such as work, clothing, housing, and education." At the beginning of the 1960s, Wolf Wolfensberger, a German-American academic, continued the drive towards Normalization. He "reworked, systematized, sociologized and generalized the concept beyond mental retardation to virtually all types of human services (Wolfensberger, 1972)."[21]

By 1990, the NHS and Community Care Act agreed that those with learning disabilities should be provided with a range of services and individual care packages tailored to suit their needs. Alongside this, suitable people were also entitled to Direct Payments which permitted them to choose the services they required. The list of services available allowed individuals the opportunity to live independently.

At the turn of the century, the white paper, *Valuing People,* was published and was the first report in thirty years that focused on learning disabilities. This guide was based on four key principles: rights, independence, choice, and inclusion. The paper outlined the new vision for people with learning disabilities with the stand-out elements being "a five-year programme to modernise local council day services"[22] and putting an end to the last long-stay hospitals.

Despite the United Kingdom changing the terminology to mental handicap in the 1990s, The United States of America continued to use stigmatising terminology until 2007. It was through the work of Dr Steven Taylor and the team he was involved in that the term mental retardation was dropped and replaced with intellectual and developmental disability.

"The term intellectual and developmental disabilities is simply less stigmatizing than mental retardation, mental deficiency, feeble-mindedness, idiocy, imbecility, and other terminology we have cast aside over the years."[23]

In March 2017, it was announced by NHS England that plans were being put into place to close Calderstones, the country's last stand-alone NHS learning disability hospital.

The Calderstones Certified Institution was initially designed to be the Sixth Lancashire County Asylum but instead, opened as the Queen Mary's Military Hospital in April 1915 during the midst of the Second World War. Once the war had ceased, the institution reopened in June 1921 as a mental health facility known as Calderstones Hospital. Despite plans to close the hospital, it continues to operate at the time of this publication, offering on-site assessments and inpatient accommodation.

Today, there is a variety of services available such as supported living, residential care, and personal support plus extended care from a range of trusts and charities. In more recent times, the learning disability and autism sector has been the centre of greater attention. "With approximately 1.5 million people in the UK with a learning disability and 1% of the population with an autism spectrum condition, it is a continuing process to make things better for those who are living with or affected by learning disability and/or autism."[24]

***

1940s *to* 1960s

"Memories of those who were associated with the hospital in war-time convoy the impression of a busy place where morale was high. Staff enjoyed life and made the best of things under the war-time conditions."

JOAN MCGRAIL

Personal Account

During the 1940s, Joan McGrail volunteered as a British Red Cross nurse at Meanwood Park Hospital. It was during this period that the institution was used as an emergency hospital to shelter and rehabilitate both British and German soldiers of World War II.

After work, I used to go to the hospital at least twice a week, 17:00 until 21:00. I would often be asked to stay late, especially when casualties were being received. This would have been from the early 1940s until I moved away from Meanwood around 1947.

Initially, I was involved with casualties who had returned from the war but as time passed, the hospital became more of a convalescence home for both soldiers and general patients from hospitals in Leeds.

The hospital was very isolated, with houses only part way up Church Lane and open fields to the other side, apart from around The Myrtle pub.

It only housed, what I describe, as young boys but as more casualties were taken in, the boys were moved elsewhere. I can recall the somewhat haunting noise and screams that many of the boys would make.

I remember that I had a tap attached to my uniform to enable me to draw water when needed. All the taps had been modified to prevent the boys from flooding the buildings.

I was in my late teens during this time so would not have been given big tasks, but I do remember washing and sterilising bandages and bedpans, talking to the soldiers and preparing bodies for the mortuary.

***

GORDON GREAVES

Personal Account

My name is Gordon James Greaves and I lived at [on] Saxon Road, Leeds from 1950-1967.

My father, Arthur James Greaves, had a landscaping business, A J Greaves, on Stainburn Avenue, Leeds and employed up to four residents from Meanwood Park Hospital for several years. They were paid 1s-2d per hour and a substantial amount of their earnings were invested in a post office account each week.

One of the men was a person of colour. He told me that his mother, who was a single parent, made false allegations against him and he ended up in Meanwood Park Hospital. It was of course very difficult having a child with two ethnicities in those days, but he was as bright as any person I have ever met. After a few years of working in our garden nursery, he told me he had hatched a plan to get out of Meanwood Park Hospital and he did. He took his girlfriend, a female resident, who was quite a character and well known in the hospital, all the way to Scotland and got married at Gretna Green. When he returned, the authorities were unable to keep them both in the hospital because they were married. I met him on a bus many years later and he told me he had four children and worked for British Rail.

For the majority of the time, we worked together without a problem but one day, while I was digging a garden border, one of the residents, for no reason, pointed his fork at me and said, "you don't think I dare do you?" And lunged at me. Had I not fallen backwards; I may not be writing this today. The thing is, he then continued working as though it had never happened.

One of the other residents who we employed was adopted by our foreman into his family but there were some family problems involving the children and he just disappeared. Some years later, I was in Minden Hospital in Germany and the same man came into my room one day to give me an injection. When he realised who I was, he pleaded with me to say nothing.

Most of the residents had very high sexual desires and we would often see two or three who had escaped, running up the middle of the ring road exposing themselves in different ways until they were caught and brought back to the hospital.

I was saddened when Meanwood Park Hospital closed and worried for many of the residents who were having to care for themselves on the outside.

***

LAUREL MACY

1969

"I remember the Down's syndrome girls being very affectionate."

It was in 1969 that Laurel Macy volunteered at Meanwood Park Hospital. "[I was] friendly with someone who had a sister in the hospital as a patient. He asked me if I would like to volunteer, so I and another friend went every Sunday afternoon for around 18 months."

Despite her friend's sister being a resident, Laurel had never stepped foot on the grounds of the hospital until her volunteering days. "I knew of its existence as I grew up in Leeds." Despite knowing of its presence, Laurel had little understanding of what the institution specialised in. "[I knew] that it was a mental hospital, but [I had] no understanding of the varied type of people it admitted. One tended to think of mental hospitals as institutions for crazy people in that era, but this was not the case."

It is important to note that Meanwood Park Hospital was not a facility for those with a mental illness. "A learning disability is not a mental illness. Learning disabilities are neurologically-based. They result from 'faulty wiring' in specific areas of the brain."[25] Where as "mental health problems can affect anyone at any time and may be overcome with treatment. A learning disability is a reduced intellectual difficulty with everyday activities which affects someone for their whole life."[26]

"[On my first day] I remember feeling a little scared but when we met the patients, the ladies, they were really lovely. Most [of them] had Down's syndrome. I can recall being shown around and we were taken to the ward with the babies in."

The ward, or villa, that Laurel brought up was in fact the Alexandra Wilson villa.

The villa was named after the first Medical Superintendent at Meanwood Park Hospital, Dr Alexander Wilson. He held the post from 1939 until his retirement in 1962. Dr Wilson was one of the few doctors in the country that specialised in the care of the mentally handicapped, establishing an out-patient clinic in mental deficiency at the Leeds University Department of Psychiatry in Hyde Terrace, Leeds, in the 1950s. He was also very influential in expanding the services of the hospital, developing the occupational facilities for the residents, establishing a School of Nursing on-site and setting up the annexe known as Crooked Acres on Spen Lane, Kirkstall. It was in May 1964 that the villa was officially opened by Dr Alexandra Wilson. Constructed as a single storey, it would accommodate forty mentally and physically handicapped children. It took on the shape of a standard 1960s school, brown stones met with large windows that spread across almost the entirety of the villa.

Laurel gave details on her first interaction with the children. "I was shocked and that's why it still stands out in my mind. Some babies had dark, thick hair all over them, some had enormous heads with tiny bodies. I have never seen anything like it and wonder what happened today when such babies are born."

The body hair that Laurel is referring to could be in fact Lanugo. "A type of fine hair that grows on the bodies of human foetuses while they are developing in the womb. These hairs disappear either by birth or shortly after when vellus hairs replace them."[27]

She confirmed that the babies she encountered were well cared for. "They were all sleeping. I am not sure how old they were or how long they had been there [but] we were told that their parents did not visit them as they could not accept that they had delivered an imperfect child. The babies with large heads had water on the brain."

Babies with large heads are a common occurrence in this book. This can be identified as either hydrocephalus or macrocephaly. With Laurel making the comment, "…had water on the brain" that possibly points towards the direction of hydrocephalus. "…[it] is a build-up of fluid in the brain. The excess fluid puts pressure on the brain, which can damage it. Many babies born with hydrocephalus (congenital hydrocephalus) have permanent brain damage."[28] It can be caused by a condition such as spina bifida"[29] which is another ailment that was common at Meanwood Park Hospital.

With the range of conditions that many of the children had, Laurel believed that many of them would have passed away before having the opportunity to grow-up.

The next villa, the one that Laurel would commence her volunteering on, was an all-female villa. "They always looked clean and the communication was relatively good. I remember the Down's syndrome girls being very affectionate. One week, I promised to bring in a magazine for one girl. The following week, I was unable to attend so I went two-weeks later. As soon as I saw her, she asked if I had remembered the magazine. Another patient seemed absolutely normal and so one day, I asked them why they were an inpatient and they [said that they were] there because of GBH (Grievous Bodily Harm.)"

During those Sunday visits, Laurel explained that the residents had a period of free time. "On a Sunday afternoon, whilst I was there, they definitely were having free time. We chatted with them and it gave them an opportunity to see familiar faces from outside the hospital. I would imagine that during the week, they were given activities and lessons."

Laurel is correct. During the week, many of the residents, depending on their ability, would go to either Industrial Therapy, Occupational Therapy or Adult Activities. These are covered later in the book.

"…I recall having long chats with the resident who was in for GBH about life in general. It was very difficult talking to patients with Down's syndrome. Although teenagers, they acted like four or five-year-olds. I can recall them being extremely affectionate and we just visited them and mixed with them for a couple of hours."

With Laurel being at the hospital during the 1960s, I asked her what the public's perception was of the place. "It was to be avoided. It was a mental asylum and once [you were] in there, you may be there for a very long time or possibly never come out. One tended to picture crazy people but I do not recall anyone like this. Cases like this were most likely in different villas. Having visited the hospital, I have positive memories of the conditions."

Based on her initial perception of Meanwood Park Hospital, Laurel's opinion had changed based on her positive experience. "[It had altered] very much. It appeared a caring, long-term institution. [It was] a large institution that looked after babies and children, caring for them well. I am sure there were adult patients there too, but I never saw them."

Laurel also believed that the residents who found home in the hospital were most suited for that environment. "Their parents, in many cases, had disowned them or could not cope with their needs. There was definitely a family feel in the areas I visited, although it was an institution."

"I finished volunteering in 1971 when I moved to London. I still volunteer now but in a hospice." The residents that Laurel worked with at Meanwood Park Hospital were unaware of her impending departure. "…I did not want to upset them. I wound down slowly when I knew I was moving away from Leeds. From once a week to once every two weeks [until] once a month. They did not seem to realise. I remember thinking that the time was right to back away. When volunteering, you get very involved."

While in London, Laurel continued to work with the physically handicapped. She admitted that she never had the opportunity to miss Meanwood Park Hospital due to her tiring schedule although now, she often thinks back to her days with the residents.

***

ROBERT SPINKS

Personal Account

In the late-1960s, into the 1970s, I was a scout leader at Roundhay Congregational Church (now St Andrew's URC).

The scout group was a thriving concern with several young and enthusiastic leaders, who, amongst other money raising activities, had speakers and turntables etc. to be able to do mobile discos. A chance meeting with one of the nursing staff of Meanwood Park Hospital secured a booking for a birthday for one of the young residents.

The disco was a raging success, with both residents and staff, from doctors to auxiliaries, but it was also a huge eye opener to some of the scouts who had come to help. They suddenly discovered that these slightly frightening people were in fact human beings who could have a good time and just like them, enjoy the music and the disco atmosphere. It was probably the first time that they saw past their disability and saw the person.

This successful evening prompted me to ask the staff if it was possible for the hospital to allow the scouts to do their voluntary service here which was a compulsory part of their scouting programme. The hospital staff were great and welcomed the boys who, in ones and twos, did their twenty-hours of service. The boys did a selection of menial tasks such as cleaning, helping in the kitchens or serving meals thus, working towards their advanced scout standard.

Little did I realise, these boys, many of them coming from somewhat privileged home lives, would form friendships and respect with people who they had not recognised as "proper" people.

This resulted in a friendly football game involving staff, residents, scouts, and scout leaders. Lacking much of the Premier League sophistication and displaying varying degrees of ability, the game further strengthened the relationship of the two parties.

I think in many ways, of all the voluntary service situations we organised for the boys, this one will live in their memory the longest. It wasn't the most exciting, it wasn't the most challenging and certainly wasn't one the boys would have chosen, but it was the one that significantly changed the way the boys thought about people with varying forms of mental illness and even as an adult, my perceptions and understanding was somewhat improved.

Now in later life, my granddaughter has some difficult issues, suffering from a rare condition (Prader-Willi syndrome) which involves some learning difficulties. I have become even more aware that some people are identified by their condition rather than by who they are. Hopefully, those boys who did their "bit" at Meanwood Park Hospital, will always see the person before the condition and will pass that insight onto their children.

***

1970s

"In 'A Hospital Plan for England and Wales' proposed in 1962, Crooked Acres was scheduled for closure, but in 1971, a change of policy in the care of the mentally handicapped favoured the provision of small units and Crooked Acres is likely to be in use for many more years."

DAVID FOSTER

1973

"I'm sure there will be someone out there who will complain, but we'd done our best and that's all we could do."

In 1971, through the help of the local council, David Foster gave up his free time during the school holidays to volunteer at various care settings. One of these was the now Thackray Medical Museum in Leeds. In 1971, the museum would have been part of St James Hospital. Along with this, Meanwood Park Hospital was another impending destination. After David returned to school, he was praised for how well he worked with children.

On the back of this praise, David approached the Meanwood Park Hospital to continue his voluntary work. "[I had] big problems finding the place because I had only been there by minibus, but I managed to find the place and meet with the voluntary organiser and started working as a voluntary worker on a Saturday."

"Then, I decided to apply for training and the course was not starting until September 1973, [this was] the Registered Nurse training course at Meanwood Park. [I] went into a group of about twelve to fifteen people and all of which were older than me. I think I was one of the youngest in the group."

Prior to David's involvement in Meanwood Park Hospital as a volunteer, he only had one other experience with the hospital. "My father told me he had once gone up to do some work in a hospital in Leeds and had gone up the drive, stopped and asked this fella for directions. He said, 'I'll take you'. He took him through some buildings, took him into a room and took out a fishing rod and started magnet fishing out of a bowl and he said he ran like hell." David did, however, have some small experience with learning disabilities. "I probably met one person with learning disabilities, a person with Down's syndrome. [She was] the sister of a friend of mine and that is the only time and I didn't even know she had a learning disability so there was nothing in schools about learning disability, nothing you would find out in the community."

David began his Registered Nurse training in 1973, qualifying in 1976. By the end of that same year, securing a full-time position at Meanwood Park Hospital was difficult. Acknowledging this, David had thought ahead and applied to work at Westwood Hospital in Bradford.

In 1860-61, The Westwood Workhouse was constructed to house 189 inmates. With the formation of the NHS in 1948, the site became known as Westwood Hospital and became a mental deficiency hospital.

On 1st January 1977, David began his role as Staff Nurse at Westwood Hospital. "The Charge Nurse had broken his leg the night before [I started] so I was thrown straight onto the ward with no Charge Nurse. I was the highest qualified staff on the ward but there were a number of experienced staff. After about 4 months, I said to the Senior Nursing Officer 'I want to be made up to Charge Nurse' and he laughed, he said 'you have only been here two minutes. If you keep on where you are, you will be made up in a year'. So, on the 1st January 1978, I became a Charge Nurse, I was about twenty-two."

After two years, David saw an advert for a Charge Nurse position at Meanwood Park Hospital. "I went for an interview, had a lousy interview, rowed all the time with the panel." After a back and forth debate, and with David seemingly not being offered the position, he was stopped on his way out and offered the post of Charge Nurse. "I started in October 1980 at Meanwood again."

On David's return to Meanwood Park Hospital, he was positioned on Villa 1 as a Charge Nurse. During this period, this villa, alongside Villa 2, was a single-storey home. "A lot of my time was basic care but what I [did was], I organised it into a sort of a group system so nurses would be responsible for a group of patients for the shift. That is not saying that someone could drop dead and they would walk over them because they are not their patient, but they would pick up that group on a morning and keep them until the end of shift. We didn't have much lifting equipment [either] because the corridors were so narrow, and we couldn't get it through the doors. [That resulted in] two people lifting and that. As I worked on there, the ward started to pick up, started getting more students. I think Norman Campbell came to us during that period and we were quite a good team, we did well. We started to change things on the ward and got the ward running correctly. I think the standard of care improved due to the hard work of the ward staff."

As one would suspect, Meanwood Park Hospital did have its own on-site mortuary although this was primarily used to store the deceased and not to conduct autopsies. "We had a few deaths on the ward. What we would do in those days is lay the body out, obviously after getting a doctor in to certify the death, call the hospital chaplain and next of kin and lay out the body. Then you'd take them on a metal trolley to the mortuary. The metal trolley was about six-foot-odd with a metal lid on it that you pull over the body. You'd put them in there and you'd wheel them down to the mortuary. You'd call the family and if they wanted to come in, they could view the body, pay their respects, and be advised on the process. They were more likely to go see them in the undertaker's chapel of rest once the undertakers had been to collect them."

Through his enthusiasm for the job and his ability to create changes for the better, David was approached to take on the role of Nursing Officer. "The job of Nursing Officer was to manage four wards in the hospital. I'd taken over Villa 1 and Villa 2 which were for people with multiple disabilities. Many of the residents were sort of more able, very able in fact, and Villa 9, I think they were more able as well. Part of the role was to manage the hospital during the day as a duty Nursing Officer and then you would be on call for the hospital as well."

In order to live at Meanwood Park Hospital, David explained that individuals had to have a learning disability and needed NHS care. Some also had physical disabilities. "From a mental health point of view, some of them did have mental health problems as well. One of the problems with mental health was there was also a reluctance from mental health services to take on people with learning disabilities because they would find that they would [have to] keep them because they needed residential care as well.

We did set up a forensic unit for people with learning disabilities towards the end of the provision at High Royds [Hospital]."

During the early period of David's career at Meanwood Park Hospital, he explained that the public's perception of the residents within the walls of the hospital was distorted. "The perception, generally, from the public was a little bit of trepidation, I think. There was a lot of confusion between learning disabilities and mental illness. Residents were seen by some members of the public as either been extremely poor souls that needed care, they need to be protected or that they were dangerous people who would come out at night and kill you, murder you or your family. For example, I was speaking to somebody after the closure who lived on the estate around Meanwood and he was telling me that every Wednesday the alarm went off at Meanwood and he would take all his washing in and his kids and run inside and he later realised that it was a fire alarm being tested on a Wednesday."

Alongside the perception of these individuals at Meanwood Park Hospital, the institution itself had a stigma attached. "To me, the idea back in probably the 70s/80s was that it was a place where people could escape from because it was a closed place, such a big place, a typical mental institution. It had a long drive, it had a bend in it, hence the term 'going around the bend', along the bend they planted a tree so you could not see beyond the bend. You could not see the mansion. It was this idea that it was a lunatic asylum, that it could be dangerous, people would avoid it. There were all sorts of those feelings, some of them quite misinformed." With these strong views circling the local community, traditionally people from the community did not enter the grounds."

Despite these perceptions, many residents did have visitors. "Some got visited quite regularly, they'd take them out into the gardens. There was a tea house run by the League of Friends. That was opened a number of times a week and it had events there. They'd take residents down to the tea house to have a drink. Some of the older residents did not understand why they were put into care and in some cases, some parents felt guilty for having put their family member into care. I've spoken to some parents who said, and this is going back years, that they'd gone to the doctors when the child was born and was told to 'get rid of it, get it in a hospital, get it in the colony' things like that. This made them feel guilty. Some residents [didn't] know why they were in there because they were just taken by their parents and left with a man. They never saw their parents again."

The residents that David cared for, across the entirety of the hospital, had a wide range of communication skills. "Even though [some] couldn't communicate verbally, you could spot changes in behaviour and they acted in their own way, to different staff, to different environments. It wouldn't be right to say that they didn't have any feelings or anything like that. They were all like little barometers, sometimes if you got to know them you could see their potential."

Meanwood Park Hospital, much like other institutions at the time, ran on a firm timetable. David attempted to alter this by adjusting the time breakfast began. "I realised why places like these institutions run like a routine. I tried to change a simple thing. I said 'I can't see why breakfast comes at 06:25/07:25, there's no need for it. Staff don't want to serve breakfast that early or [the residents don't want] their breakfast at that time. So, I tried to get them to bring it later and it caused such a problem because the night staff wanted to get residents up and I didn't want them to get them up so they thought they'd done something wrong. What we found is that if we tried to do the breakfasts later, then it put every villa out on the whole block because they got theirs later as well. Then once they didn't get theirs on time, they rushed to get their people out. [They] then came to get the [food] trolleys and the trolleys weren't ready on time. So, from me trying to change it on my ward, I upset the whole hospital, nearly caused a riot."

After breakfast, residents who had activities planned for the day were sent on their way. For those who didn't, David allowed them to remain in bed for a short while. They would return for lunch before returning to their earlier activities. In the evenings, residents were allowed free-time. "I think if you measured what they were doing in the hospital at night and during the day against people with learning disabilities out in the community, you'd probably find they had more activities than those outside."

David went on to explain the suitability of the villas that he worked on. "Today, they wouldn't be fit for purpose. These places were built at a specific time, in specific, social and political conditions."

In Industrial Therapy, residents would fulfil small contracts for local businesses and earn a small wage. Most were menial and involved either sorting an assortment of small objects or connecting pieces together. Originally, Industrial Therapy was the focus of psychiatric hospitals. Phillippe Pinel, a French physician, and William Tuke, an English Quaker, began the Moral Treatment movement. They questioned society's beliefs regarding the mentally ill. Pinel introduced work treatment for the insane. He believed that "moral treatment meant treating one's emotions and using occupation as a way to direct their minds away from emotional disturbances."[30] Pinel followed this up by integrating literature, music and physical exercise to improve emotional stress. This soon made its way into similar institutions with the aim of educating, improving life skills and organisation skills to name a few. In places like Meanwood Park Hospital, it allowed those who saw the institution as their home, to go out and work.

"As a student I had to work in there. One of the contracts I worked on was bubble tops, the things you put on bubbles. The problem is, when they didn't meet their contracts, the staff would have to work on the job to get the contracts done."

Another daily occurrence for residents was physiotherapy. Based on site, this was headed by Superintendent Physiotherapist Terry Craig. One of the most interesting aspects of physiotherapy was rebound therapy. This programme makes use of trampolines to improve balance, coordination and motor skills while also being a pleasurable activity. The suggestion of using trampolines in special education came about in the 1950s but was further developed by Eddy Anderson who worked with both physical and learning disabilities.

Despite the wealth of on-site activities, efforts were also made to take residents out of the hospital and down to the coast for holidays. Popular destinations were Torquay, Skegness, Scarborough, and Cornwall. "Obviously, there was a lot of staring [from the public.] I remember being at Scarborough on the beach and it was almost like a crocodile coming over the sand on a boiling hot day and it was people with learning disabilities because they looked like they were in a school party, like a long crocodile and we all had boots on. You could always tell, [they had] these hospital issued parkas with the fur collars, all marching around the beach, that didn't help. We gradually started to do smaller group day trips."

In the early years of Meanwood Park Hospital, residents, or patients as they were originally referred as, would most likely remain in the hospital until their passing. It was the change in terminology that rebranded these types of institutions as homes, referring to those living in them as residents. "I don't think they saw it as a hospital, I think they saw it as where they lived. It was their life and it's what they did, but they had nothing to compare it with. I can remember somebody who had been admitted under the 1913 Mental Health Act as a moral defective. She had a child out of wedlock and had been put in there. When I trained, I was trained for the care of the mentally subnormal and that term changed. They were [then] known as severely subnormal [and then] to mental handicap. But the idea of low grades and high grades, that was a term I didn't like. At the end of the day, they were people, sometimes they were even friends." It would be at the end of the 1990s before the terminology saw another change, replacing mental handicap with learning disability.

The term high-grades and low-grades is one that continually appeared in each interview. This most likely originated from the early years of the hospital, back when it was known as Meanwood Park Colony. Patients who were deemed very able and capable of looking after themselves, were often required to assist other residents with personal hygiene and feeding. This, as one could imagine, created a hierarchy. The label, unfortunately, stuck throughout Meanwood Park Hospital's operation. Attempts were made to expel this term but through long-stay residents and old-school staff, it remained. It is important to note that during David's time, other residents weren't made to assist.

"There was this ward, I won't mention the ward, but every day the chap on there, let's call him Arthur, he would make the tea for all the staff and they would say 'Arthur, bring two cups, we'll have tea.' He would go back and forth every day for years and then one day, the Charge Nurse had another visitor. Arthur had gone to the kitchen to make the teas, he walked into the kitchen and Arthur was peeing in the teapot and he's done it for years. That was the way he got his own back for running back and forth as a skivvy. He never made tea again."

David went on to explain that 99% of people in Meanwood were informal patients. Much like today, residents were either brought into the hospital voluntarily or involuntarily. "In theory, they could walk off anytime they liked [but] we had a duty of care to bring them back." During one-night shift, confusion came about due to the villa enforcing locked doors. "On one of the wards, the day staff went off and handed over to the night staff. Now what you're supposed to do was go round and touch everybody practically and see anybody you've got worries about and introduce them to the night staff and I would always insist that. On this particular night they did that, and this was an agency nurse, she'd come on and had been introduced to all the patients. She locked all the doors and started to make the coffee. Someone had walked in the kitchen and said 'can you open the door? I want to go' and she said, 'no love, go sit down and I'll bring you a coffee.' 'No, I want to go.' 'Sit down and I'll bring you some coffee.' 'You can't keep me here.' So, she got on the phone and called the night Charge Nurse who came across and he said, 'that's not a patient, that's a relative, you've locked a relative in.'

It wasn't only relatives who were being mistaken for residents. "I could blend in as a patient really and people actually said that they couldn't tell the difference between patients and staff. When I was a Nursing Officer, I would work until 10pm sometimes and I would go on the wards and see the night staff. I would walk onto a ward and the lights would be dimmed and the nurses station would stand up and it happened a few times and one night I said, 'don't stand up for me' and one nurse said 'I'm not standing up in reverence for you, I'm standing up so you can see me.' That was a big deflate for me, I thought they were standing up because I was the Nursing Officer." In the early days, the only item of clothing that allowed staff to be identified, if worn, was their white coat or nursing uniform. As a student in 1973, another option was a hospital issued suit but unfortunately for David, they weren't in stock. "They didn't have any of those, but they did have some donkey jackets left. It was a short jacket, white trousers. When I walked on the children's ward, they all thought it was the ice cream man returning so I got rid of that after a while. I couldn't work with white coats with long sleeves, so I cut them off and had short sleeves."

With the aim to be self-sustained, Meanwood Park Hospital had numerous facilities. Some that survived the hospital's transition through time, others being left behind. "It was built as a colony, so it was supposed to be self-contained. At one time, it had its own gardens, workshops, and kitchens. As the hospital gradually ran down, other services came on site who could not be housed elsewhere. We had an education department and school, we had Getaway Girls, they are still around today, they came on for a time. It had its own tuck shop and its own theatre for dental extractions."

During David's time, behavioural drugs were a common occurrence. "The major sort of behavioural drugs was chlorpromazine, thioridazine, haloperidol, lithium sodium, lithium carbonate."

An intellectual disability cannot be treated by medication. There is no cure, but early involvement can lessen their effects, allowing these individuals to develop ways to cope with their disability. Despite this, medication was commonly in use at Meanwood Park Hospital. It was primarily used to treat the challenging behaviours associated with a learning disability.

"My experience with them was that consultants would always prescribe what they were comfortable with. They did not go wild and prescribe things that they did not have knowledge in."

Haloperidol is in fact a typical antipsychotic medication, but it can be used in the treatment of a variety of conditions. One of those being agitation which is thought to be one of the most common forms of psychological distress for people with learning disabilities.

Meanwood Park Hospital did in fact have its own dispensary on Villa 3. As the years progressed and with the introduction of a new pharmacist from Seacroft, medication became more tailored to the resident's individual needs.

Many of the residents continued to receive state benefits while housed in Meanwood Park Hospital with countless individuals banking a large sum of money. "I actually served on the patients' money committee and my drive was to try and get them to spend money. Rather than having nothing, which is a crime, having £1000 in the bank was a crime as well because it was doing nothing for them. If we bought them proper clothes, good clothes, you couldn't send it to the laundry because you'd get it back like dolls clothes, so they were washed on the ward and we tried to separate them out. We would only send hospital issued stuff to the hospital laundry. Hospital issued clothing in my time had patients' names inside them. In fact, if you lost anybody you would just say 'look in the collar'. The only time it came unstuck was while we were in Bradford. We found someone had absconded and they had taken someone else's clothes."

Towards the late-1980s, with the drive towards community care beginning to creep in, David was asked if he would take on a position in the community. "They wanted someone to run it. Community to me and a lot of people was the star job of the whole lot because you are out there in the community, managing community nurses plus there were twelve community homes and about five other group homes as well so you were managing a very large part of the service. Then, we got a new Unit General Manager. I then became a Clinical Unit Manager for Meanwood Park which was part of my clinical unit plus community nurses, plus group homes as well."

At the same time, David was honest with his staff about the imminent future. "I told them the truth, I told them exactly how it was going to go. We wanted to avoid redundancies because we wanted to keep every member of staff we could, everybody had a place really."

To help with the closure of Meanwood Park Hospital, the resettlement team was involved in planning the next steps of deinstitutionalization. "We couldn't take all people with learning disabilities through to the next stages because there wasn't a big enough NHS provision. Although some people did need social care, they could go and live in ordinary houses with care staff so other providers came in and tended to take on some of these services. We then had to work out who would go to social care and who would stay with the NHS and to stay within the NHS, they would literally ask for the reasons why they were to remain and not move into social care. But gradually, they were moving some of the more able people out. But the more time you spend in hospital, the more institutionalised you get. It's very difficult to take someone from a hospital and put them straight into the community and expect them to survive."

Feelings amongst the residents were mixed. Many of them saw Meanwood Park Hospital as their home, others were unaware of what was transitioning around them.

In the final days at Meanwood Park Hospital, David began clearing out vacant villas. Removing furniture that would later be auctioned off to local businesses. "We gave stuff away to schools; we gave things away to the Thackray Museum. We had a truck come from Slovakia to collect a load of beds. They came without any sort of tail lift and drove to the hospital on a Friday night at about 4pm and we had to help him load this long, massive trailer full of beds. He couldn't speak a word of English and he had no tail lift, so we had to cart each one on. I was able to give him directions to Shipley where he had to go next in pigeon German."

With the amount of outside presence increasing, it led to an array of unusual situations. "I got called in one afternoon as there were noises coming from the unit under HQ. I said, 'get the police, I'm going to go down there and sort it out.' I got in my car and I drove as fast as I could. While I was getting out the car I could hear a lot of banging going on and as I got to the door, this fella came out with a boiler on his back, he must have been 6ft 10 with a big black beard and a boiler suit. He saw the look on my face, the look on my face was absolute shock and horror, the size of this fella. He had a boiler on his back, that's how big he was, a big copper boiler, and he said 'it's alright, I've been asked by one of the engineers to pick it up' and as he said that, the police came. I learned from this that I should not charge into situations."

"I had to throw off a Channel 4 film crew because they were on the drive taking pictures of the building. They were trying to portray the closure as another hospital closure by the government. I came down and asked them who had given them permission to film on site. When they said nobody, I said, 'you better get off site' and when they didn't move, I stuck my groin in the camera, 'film this.' They got the message and moved off site."

"I remember coming in after being on holiday and it was a Friday night. I'd left some papers in the mansion and it had gotten to the stage where we had moved the switchboard out to the back of the mansion, and it closed at night, so it was locked up. I went to grab some papers, took my daughter, brought them out and the next day we'd found out that the place had been broken into and the robbers had been stashed in the cellar waiting for it to get dark to open the safe at night but they hadn't found anything."

The furniture that remained was to be broken down and David, along with other members of staff, spent their final day at Meanwood Park Hospital doing just that. "We had this massive skip outside and we were bouncing up and down trying to break up chairs to get rid of them and I remember they were having a board meeting in the mansion and they were looking out of the window watching us jump up and down in this skip, thinking we were mad, saying that we'd lost it again. We made sure every ward had been cleared and we made sure there were no records left behind. We were relieved that we had got it to the finish line, and I think we'd done fairly well. I'm sure there will be someone out there who will complain, but we'd done our best and that's all we could do."

Residents moved out in phases, many of them entering the community. Those who didn't find themselves in community homes were cared for in Woodland Square at St Mary's Hospital in Armley, Leeds. "The idea was to provide a range of provisions that would carry on NHS services in Leeds, so it has specific reasons. It would house some with challenging behaviours but there would also be an assessment unit for people passing through and a respite care unit. So, there were bungalows which would take people with severe learning disabilities and they also acquired houses for people with challenging behaviour as well. We had a system where people could move through the system. They could come into the assessment unit and either return home or as a last resort, move into a residential home if there were provision and they were deemed to need NHS or social services care."

The community bungalows that Meanwood Park Hospital utilised were specifically constructed for them. "In the project office, we used to get objections from some local resident groups. Prior to building the home or before moving in, we used to speak to the local community, local MPs and especially councillors. One councillor in general, they had all sorts of objections about how one of the bungalows would increase traffic in their area, ambulances would be coming up all day bringing people, yet they came and opened the place."

It was in 1997, the same year as the closure of Meanwood Park Hospital that David was offered a managerial role at St Mary's Hospital. A position in which he held for just over a year. Through redundancy, he moved into the private sector in Harrogate before returning to Leeds as a Service Manager at a local charity.

Before the interview ended, David offered some of his memorable moments at Meanwood Park Hospital.

"There was the recreation hall which I had to go on call to see it burn down. It became a store for Moortown Furnishings, and we had an electrical fault back in the 80s and it burned down, I took my daughter and she loved it."

"I got a call one night from a ward on the weekend. They said, 'we've heard a big bang.' One of the patients had just come back from being out. 'He's got a gun, what do we do?' Now, nobody ever wrote a manual to tell you what to do if someone has a gun, so I said, 'have you got the gun?' 'Yes.' 'Call the police.' 'Shouldn't we tell his father or something, his father brought him back, he could be a bank robber.' We called the police, and they came out and they examined it and it was a starting pistol. What had happened was, his father had been doing a race and he had a starting pistol. He put it in the glove compartment of the car. When he stopped at the garage to get some petrol on his way back to the hospital, his son had gone into the glove compartment and put it in his pocket and took it back to the hospital."

"I was called in one night to say horses were running around the site, so I got in the car with my daughter and went up. As we got there, the police were blocking the gate off and I said 'I've come to round up the horses' and they said 'no you're not, you're not touching them. There's a mare and its foal running round like mad.' So, the staff brought all the residents in and locked all the wards, and the horses were just running around the site so I said, 'can I do anything?' And he said, 'yes, go to the top gate and block it.' I went and blocked it with the car and sat there for about half an hour. Some of the horses came towards me and they just managed to shim down the side of my car and straight back down Tong Lane. I got in my car and we drove backwards down Tong Lane chasing them and back through the front gate and back up into the grounds again and past the coppers. I went back up to the top gate and blocked the gate and then about an hour later, a police woman had been called in to round them up and as she was rounding them up, I went to pat one of them and it stood right on my foot. They managed to take them out of the ground. I then saw a small police car, they were loading this old fella into the back, he was the owner of the horses and he tethered them on some land illegally and they had just run off. I used to get called in for loads of daft things."

David had more than twenty-five years of experience at Meanwood Park Hospital, seeing the evolution of care unfold in front of him and in some cases, contributing ideas and theories that would improve the health and overall outlook of the residents. "[These hospitals] were a product of an era and I find it very difficult to criticize the era because that's that they believed, that's what they wanted and that was the general philosophy. What it does tell us though is that their product of ideology is a very strong ideology. It worked. It was something that guided care and people believed in it. I won't criticize the past and we should learn from it and in times of economic problems and lack of money, it could come back again quite easily."

"It was an institution, and it provided a service at that moment in time, but it became outdated in the mid-20th century. It served its purpose when it was built with its philosophies and its ideologies but over time, philosophies changed, and the ideologies changed."

"I always have a lot of respect for people who worked in Meanwood because most of them generally cared [about] what they were doing. They did want to see good care. I'll always give them credit for the caring side of it. We always get people who stand out as being better or worse, luckily the worst ones were only a minority and I generally believe most people did care."

***

AMELIA BROWN

1975

"It was their home; however, it was not home like."

It would be in East Berlin where Amelia Brown had her first role as a "Mother's help", a local term used to describe an individual who works or lives with a family and takes on the family's responsibility for childcare and housework. She carried out this role with a diplomat's family for nine months before moving to Leeds to work as a noodle-packer at Rakusen's.

"I wanted to work with people and help them in some way. I thought I might like to train as a nurse, and I was interested in helping people with learning difficulties or mental handicap as it was called. My younger sister had mild learning difficulties."

Meanwood Park Hospital was a slight mystery to Amelia at the time. The first time she encountered the institution was during her initial interview. "I had [never] been there but I knew about it. I think I had heard positive things. The people who interviewed me were nice. They knew I wouldn't be staying long as I was thinking of applying to become a nurse. Some of the people I saw in the grounds seemed a bit strange, dressed in odd clothes. [They were] ill fitting, shapeless. The grounds were nice, and the villa system seemed cosier than a big hospital."

During her short stay at the hospital, Amelia worked on Villa 7 which she described as being an all-female home. "Women slept in a big dormitory upstairs. They had a bed and bedside cupboard each. We got them up and washed and dressed if they needed help. We then served breakfast and helped some of them eat. Some helped with the tasks such as making beds and laying tables etc. They were called high-grades and low-grades depending on their ability. Some went to Industrial Therapy where I remember them packing pencils. The next group went to Occupational Therapy. Some stayed on the ward and we looked after them."

When it came to personal hygiene, a majority of the staff followed a routine of helping residents to bath and shower rather than providing bedside washes. "The bathrooms were functional rather than pleasant."

In regard to the condition of Villa 7, Amelia explained that the Sister in charge enforced rules to keep the villa running like a hospital and not like their home which, to some, it was their home, it was all they had ever known. "Some would impose petty rules. They would stop people going out to the bingo in the evening and send them to bed for being cheeky. Everyone was kept clean, well fed and the bed linen was changed. There was also a lot of love and care from most of the staff for the residents or patients I think they were called."

This behaviour was seemingly mirrored on other villas with some staff cutting corners. "I remember one member of staff on another villa mixed the patients main course and pudding together as he thought it made no difference."

The residents who stayed behind, the ones who were either unable to participate due to their disability level or were merely too elderly, would most likely be taken for a walk around the grounds or remain within their villa. "There were musical instruments [that were] stored in cupboards but not used, so some of us Nursing Assistants did singing and music." To further improve the residents' day, Amelia and the other nursing assistant on shift were able to assemble a collection of paint. "We painted and put the pictures on the walls, but the Sister took them down as it was a hospital."

On Villa 7, Amelia cared for an assortment of characters, some that may have been able to live outside of the institution, maybe not independently but undoubtedly with some assistance. "Nobody should have lived there but some were definitely in the wrong place, I used to read the files."

Some of the residents who were more able, the ones most likely to flourish in the community may have found themselves at Crooked Acres, the annexe on Spen Lane which remained in use during Amelia's time. "I remember one woman who later moved to Crooked Acres, she had a boyfriend and they used to meet up. It was a true romance and they both moved to Chapel Allerton."

Nevertheless, many of the residents housed in Meanwood Park Hospital did suffer from a range of learning and physical disabilities. "Some of them didn't speak. One had severe epileptic fits and the one who was profoundly deaf had no one to communicate with on the villa."

In the mid-1970s, amenities at the hospital were sparse. Amelia was only able to remember the League of Friends tearoom plus the central laundry and kitchen. "The clothes were often communal and kept in a store and sent to the laundry on site, but some had clothes with their names on, possibly the ones who had visitors." Despite a lack of activities being available on site, efforts were made to take residents away from the hospital. "They did get some money because when we went on trips, they got money to spend. I don't remember ever clothes shopping with them, but I went on day trips. We once went to the seaside at Filey I think and once to Blackpool for the [Christmas] lights and fish and chips. It was nice for them to go out somewhere new, but we were a big group and people stared at us and made comments."

To Amelia's knowledge, the public's perception of those with learning disabilities in the 1970s was not generally positive. "It was not very acceptable to be out and about. Nobody was horrible but one group of German teenagers at the seaside were mocking them and were very shocked when I told them off in German. We could only go to the pub with a few who seemed most 'normal' and could fit in."

True to her word, Amelia left Meanwood Park Hospital just six months later. "I was sad to leave the people, but I knew it wasn't somewhere I wanted to stay as I knew it wasn't the right way. But as a nursing assistant, you were powerless, and you just had to fit in with the system. Some [residents] were upset [that I was leaving] but I did go back to visit, and I went on some trips with them. I stayed in touch a bit with the lady who went to Crooked Acres. I was glad when it closed but sad that there are so many hospitals for people with learning disabilities as they should not exist."

"It was not a suitable environment for people to live their whole lives. It was their home; however, it was not home like. The hospital system with nurses, Sisters, uniforms, and the rigidity of the routines was all wrong for these people. The villas allowed little privacy or individuality. It did not afford them dignity. They had no say over their lives. I guess it did give a place where they were accepted but they were cut off from the outside world."

"I learnt a lot. It made me determined to study and train so that I could have some say in making things better. I did have some nice times but mostly I felt that it offered too little to the people who lived there."

***

GRACE JONES

1976

"I don't know how to be a carer without caring, bonding is to care."

Despite commencing her volunteer work in 1976, Grace Jones was introduced to Meanwood Park Hospital in the 1960s, aged between twelve to fifteen. One of her childhood friends had lived in the farmhouse that occupied the grounds of the hospital. "We were just school friends hanging about, so I got to know the patients."

Grace's friend had explained to her that the farmhouse belonged to the hospital which allowed many of the residents to work there, growing and harvesting food for the hospital. "The farm was at the end where Penny Field School is. It was a vegetable farm; the food was for the kitchens."

The farmland that Grace noted was tended to by the residents c.1935. "Fifty-six acres of market gardens were worked by men who lived at the hospital to produce potatoes, oats and vegetables for Meanwood Park and other hospitals."[31] Rather than working on the farm, I believe the patients tended to the gardens during the 1960s with Dr Douglas Spencer's jubilee notes indicating this.

"They had parties there for Valentine's Day, Halloween, Christmas and I got invited along with my friend, as were her parents. As a child, I was told it was a colony of nutters, so I thought that everyone would be tied up in bed so I was surprised to find that they were people who could walk and talk."

It would be in 1976 that Grace began her volunteer work which was simply offering companionship to the residents. "It was just chatting to the patients, playing with the children, talking about their lives. Occasionally, going to the local pubs; Bay Horse and The Myrtle."

Her volunteer work allowed her to rotate through the various villas of Meanwood Park Hospital, one of those being the Alexandra Wilson villa. "I worked on the villa with school age children, but I also worked on the baby villa which I hated, AW. There were about twenty babies all with special needs crawling about just wanting someone to pick them up and love them. There was never enough staff. The odd baby did [have physical deformities], there were a few [with] Down's syndrome and ill babies with cystic fibrosis. I remember a baby with hydrocephalus. They had hundreds of toys and games but sometimes only two staff were on. Times were taken up by feeding, changing, and pushing prams around the park but that took up a lot of time for two staff and twenty babies. Some were ill so that took up a lot of time. The villa was said to accommodate forty babies but not while I was there. Staff were ill trained, not like today [where] you have to go on lots of courses before you can work with learning disabilities."

"[The children weren't] given real diagnoses. [They were known as] imbeciles, retards and the feeble-minded. Mainly, it was said that they were mentally retarded. Care workers were not privileged to read care plans like we do today. But also, [they were] called high-grades and low-grades. I don't think the children should have been at Meanwood, I didn't think anyone should have but I think people of that time were ignorant to mental health. People outside of the hospital knew nothing of the patients so everyone I spoke to thought it was the best place for them and it was keeping us (the public) safe. Some staff who worked at the hospital couldn't care less about the patients or their needs while others thought some of the residents had been wrongly admitted and shouldn't have been there in the first place. I asked someone why they had put their child in there and they said that the doctor said to them, 'think of a barrel of apples, if you get a rotten one you get rid of it' and they did. He wasn't the first person to say something to me like that. One person told me that they wanted to keep their son at home, but the doctors insisted they would be better off there. Once the hospital started to let family and friends visit, they came to the hospital every week. [Previously], they could not visit. Apparently you had to get permission but someone in the hospital was found to have been physically abused and the family of that person were lawyers or something like that and organised some sort of parent group and things changed."

As previously mentioned, despite being a hospital for those with learning disabilities, Meanwood Park Hospital did take on individuals with dual diagnoses hence Grace mentioning the ignorance towards mental health in the 1970s.

Prior to the children going to Penny Field School, the hospital did have an on-site Department of Education, a large building that sat between Villa 10 and 11. It was constructed with a small courtyard in the centre. As children were gradually restricted from being admitted to the hospital, a new purpose-built school, Penny Field, was constructed.

Another villa that Grace volunteered on was Villa 1. "[This] was classed as the lowest grade possible, the 'dregs' as it was known as. It was for people with the most physical, and what was thought to be, the most mentally unbalanced."

This villa, alongside its neighbour Villa 2, was used to house those with mobility problems. They were constructed to the far north-west of the grounds and faced onto the woodland. Both homes were single storey to allow access for wheelchair users.

Grace's volunteer work at Meanwood Park Hospital continued for roughly a year before she was employed by the hospital as a domestic. "[I] mopped the villas. I was what you called a 'floater' so didn't have a villa designated to me. [Also], washing up and anything that nobody else would do but I got the chance to talk to lots of people."

"People with Tourette's, people telling me that they had family and just got left there, people saying that they had babies but had them taken off them, people telling me they were there so they could be with people like themselves. Men asking to have sex with me and people asking me to buy cigarettes for them. One resident, who was Jewish, told me they loved eating Jewish bacon and that they were a 'dirty Jew.' Another resident, also Jewish, told me they had regular sex on the field with another resident. In 1993, I had the pleasure to work with both Jewish residents when the Jewish Welfare Board got them out when the hospital closed. There was one resident who walked about all day collecting bits of string, they carried this huge ball of string everywhere. There was also a resident who had a huge head and a tiny body like the doll that was in fashion once. They were so disabled, and they were pushed about in a huge pram. There used to be large bins where the waste food was put, and some patients climbed in and out for food. Once, when I was looking out of the window, a naked man ran across the field and I told the other staff. Their reply was, 'was it a patient or staff?' It did get me thinking about who I was working with."

It was a pleasant transition into the role of domestic for Grace and despite thoroughly enjoying her position, after two years she became a care assistant. It was her time spent as a volunteer that encouraged her to return to a more hands-on role. "I've always been a caring person."

Keeping with the traditional role of a 'floater', Grace moved amongst the villas, providing care for a range of residents. The home in which she enjoyed the most was Villa 12. This was an all-male villa with the residents having challenging behaviour. "Most men were very chatty. They told me about their lives, and I was told by staff that some of the men had been put there because they had raped women but mainly, they asked me to bring books or pens. One resident told me where they had [previously] lived and that they had been put there for no reason. They asked me to find out where their family was. I know I shouldn't have but I did find his family. They told me to mind my own business and wanted nothing to do with them as they were a 'spastic'. I never told them this, but it made me both angry and sad."

Grace's least favourite placement was the Alexandra Wilson villa. "[There were] not enough staff to give the babies affection which of course was not allowed anyway, it was not considered part of your role as the child could form a bond with you and you might never go on that villa again. I am a caring person and over the years I've been told hundreds of times not to hug people, don't invade space, things could look sexual, I don't know how to be a carer without caring, bonding is to care."

By 1983, seven years after she began, Grace fell pregnant and left her role as a care assistant. "I was really sad to leave Meanwood Park. [I had] known it since I was 12. I went on to be a dinner lady at our local school to work around my children's needs and then onto home care. I then went to work in a residential home for learning disabilities run by Leeds Jewish Welfare Board, working with eight of the patients from Meanwood Park for thirteen years. I then went to work for Leeds Mencap for eleven years. I now work for Royal Mencap."

"I liked it there. I never saw any physical abuse, but I heard it went on. There was a lack of understanding for what to do with people with learning disabilities and everyone was led to believe it was better for them to be there. Also, it was safer for us to lock up someone who might hurt you or your family. People used to have large families and had no knowledge how to cope. When the hospital closed, some of the patients found themselves at a complete loss, they didn't know how to cook, shop and they were thrown into the unknown. They felt lost without all the people they had grown up with. As a Mother, I would have never let my child or family member go into Meanwood Park. Babies would have thrived better with a mum but then again, lots of mums don't look after their children as they should. Maybe if the staff there had been trained properly the abuse would not have gone on or if the main people had done their job properly people could have thrived."

"I loved working there and I loved the patients. I felt that I made a difference. I learnt so much about people. My greatest attribute is that I care, it's also my greatest downfall.

I was upset to leave, if it had not been for family circumstances and it was still open, I would still be there."

***

SARAH READ

1977

"Meanwood Park Hospital was never needed. There is no reason to exclude people from the community."

Unlike many of my interviewees, Sarah Read had already gained her general nursing qualification prior to starting at Meanwood Park Hospital. To continue her development, she undertook a conversion course that allowed her to move into the field of learning disabilities. On completion, Sarah was an Enrolled Nurse for the Mentally Handicapped.

Despite being newly qualified, Sarah had already been introduced to Meanwood Park Hospital six years prior through a further education course. She undertook a placement at the hospital over a period of twelve months.

"At first I was shocked and scared but after a short while, I saw individuals with personalities."

During her twelve-month placement at the hospital, Sarah was assigned to the activities centre and the Alexandra Wilson villa, a period of six months in each.

The activities centre was more tailored to residents who were unable to participate in Occupational Therapy or Industrial Therapy. The aim of these activities was to improve the individuals motor skills and problem-solving skills as well as increasing their self-esteem.

At the time, Sarah was unaware of their diagnoses but reflecting on the situation now, she explained that they most likely had a profound or severe learning disability. "At that time, I was 16/17 and I thought that Meanwood looked after them and that maybe they couldn't live outside but I quickly learnt that the support they needed could be provided outside in the community."

The Alexandra Wilson villa remained consistent throughout the 1970s, housing children with both physical and learning disabilities. "I think most of the children were teenagers or thereabouts. The building was modern compared to the rest of the hospital. It had a large dining room come lounge and a couple of large bathrooms. The bedrooms had about six people in and I think there were three of these and a couple of single rooms. It was a large one storey building with a large garden. I just remember lots of large cots and feeding everyone pea green mush. I went on a Friday, always fish."

Most, if not all the children on the villa, slept in cots specifically tailored to mean their physical needs. These are designed much like a regular cot but are sized to meet the dimensions of a single bed. Cots for disabilities have progressed significantly since the days of Meanwood Park Hospital, with today's making use of padded sides to prevent injury. The ones in use at the hospital and even at other institutions around the world were constructed with metal railings, no protective sides and sometimes, a steel cover to prevent the child from leaving the crib. Rather than being used as a method of confinement, these top coverings prevented the individual dropping from a height which could cause a significant injury.

Unlike a volunteer, Sarah had a more hands-on role when it came to patient care. "I assisted wherever. I helped with washing and dressing, feeding, taking them to school or helping with laundry."

Despite spending twelve months at the hospital, Sarah's perception went unchanged. "[It was] a cold sort of place [in winter]. Feeding pea green mush to children who I didn't know how to relate to, and no one showed me, I just improved my laundry folding skills."

Sarah returned to Meanwood Park Hospital in 1983 as an Enrolled Nurse and immediately noticed a difference in the running of the institution. "The most obvious one was the mixing of men and women on some of the villas as before they had been segregated on opposite sides of the hospital."

Despite having some previous experience with the Alexandra Wilson villa, Sarah was employed to work on Villa 4, an all-female villa for individuals with mild to moderate learning disabilities. "It was as homely as we could [make it] but the ladies still slept in dormitories and shared bathrooms with little privacy. [It had a] large dining room and lounge area."

"We had a few younger ladies who were more learning disabled but most could have been more independent if they had not lived at Meanwood. Often when they spoke, they spoke of how they became residents, and they showed their dissatisfactions with the life they could have had. One lady was admitted after becoming pregnant and when a staff member's daughter became pregnant at 16, we all knitted and bought presents. She became upset and said, 'that's what happened to me and look where I ended up, no one knitted for me.' One resident had run away down south as they were fed up with their dad. When they were returned home, they had them admitted to Meanwood. They swore blind that they would have made it down south."

Sarah's day had not changed much from when she was on placement, she continued to assist with personal hygiene and ensuring residents were on time to their daily activities. Those who didn't attend any activities, remained on the villa. "Some had retired, and they had been classed as working girls in the past, working in various places such as laundry, kitchens and the children's villa."

With closure not being envisioned at that moment, many of the residents were lasting fixtures of the hospital. "Slowly over time they passed away before being offered a chance to move on."

After twelve months, Sarah was transferred to Villa 7, a two-storey home for female adults. She found that change was more acceptable here compared to that of Villa 4 which she described as having a very institutional approach. "[It was] easier to bring about change [as we had] younger staff. People [were] willing to move along and give a higher quality of care, more progressive. We also asked questions and involved them in plans and choices, individually and as a group."

"One lady kept messing with the radio when she was transferred from another villa. She would turn all the knobs and it took us a while to realise that she didn't like pop music but loved classical music, so we set up a music system for her in another room. She had no speech [so was unable to verbally communicate]."

In 1994/5, after short stretches on other villas, Sarah was moved to the Assessment and Treatment Unit (ATU). By then, the closure of Meanwood Park Hospital had been decided, with the drive towards community care in full motion. These units were designed to provide short-term care for individuals with learning disabilities before moving back into the community. Despite the aim of short-term care, many individuals are known to have been homed in them for years.

"[It was] a new challenge, everything was changing. I worked with people who had been identified as needing social care and I wasn't sure if I wanted to leave health care, so I transferred to a new unit. [It was used] to assess and treat people with learning disabilities who lived in the community and had [suffered] a crisis. Maybe [they had] mental health issues or maybe their care provision had broken down. The length of stay varied from weeks to months, most were fine but occasionally, someone would be admitted very mentally unwell with an acute illness including a psychotic episode. Others arrived a little unkempt and needed some care."

It was interesting to learn from Sarah that despite having a psychotic episode or having a diagnosed mental illness, they weren't cared for in a psychiatric institution such as High Royds Hospital which was just 7.5 miles from Meanwood Park Hospital. They were cared for at the ATU due to their learning disability being more of a priority.

"We worked hard to maintain their usual routine and [that they] attended their usual day-care. The first few days would be on the unit as they were assessed with a baseline medical test completed. Some patients had an individual support worker, and they came to work as usual with their client. Each person's plan and care were very individual so [there was] no set routine. It was a safe place for vulnerable people to access support. It was a very serious unit. [It] developed as changes were happening to the whole of learning disabilities. It was the future, not long-term care, [it was] very short term with a purpose. [It had] individual care plans [and had] more qualified nurses, intense at times. We also continued into the community, [providing] care and support if needed."

With Meanwood Park Hospital entering its final days, the ATU was moved to St Mary's Hospital. "We had all worked there for a long time, but it was time for change and improvement." The service users who were present at the assessment unit were also transferred to St Mary's Hospital but their stay, as planned, was short-term. "They came with us, but they were not long-stay patients. They had come into the assessment unit a few weeks before [but] they all had homes in the community."

"[It was] lovely working in the community with a small group of people [and] giving person-centred care." Despite her enjoyment, Sarah moved on to work for a non-profit organization, shifting from an inpatient environment to home-based care.

"Meanwood Park Hospital was never needed. There is no reason to exclude people from the community. I think it provided a safe place and families liked the idea their loved ones were safe. I think there was a lot of unkindness and some staff behaving in a 'I'm better than you' way. Maybe, slowly through education, the powers that be finally saw that the community was the place. It's still not perfect, just look at reported hate crimes against people with learning disabilities, but it is better than exclusion."

"I loved it, the opportunity to change people's lives for the better, to encourage independence and self-worth and to see people be able to make choices for themselves. Also, [I felt] sadness that they were not valued or treated with dignity."

***

1980s *to* 1990s

"On 28 November, a turf cutting ceremony was performed by Councillor Jim McKenna to start building work on the new £1.6 million PLD core unit designed by Harrogate Architects HMA, Senior Partner Philip Montgomery, at St Mary's Hospital."

MARGARET HARTLEY

Personal Account

I started work in about 1980 (or late 1970s) as a secretary in the Nurse's Home and I went to St James's Hospital for the interview. It was not far from where we lived so I could walk to work.

It was the first building on the drive. A couple of other ladies worked in that office too and we became good friends. The boss used to bring his dog into work, it was a small spaniel. Sometimes, he would ask if I could take it for a walk, but I would need a strong stomach. One day, he thought he would try to be clever by dictating a letter in German, but I could speak German. He was a very good boss though and when my father was ill in hospital in Sheffield, he told me to take a day off to go see him. He did not ask me to, he told me to.

It was the best job I ever had, I really enjoyed it. It was a nice place to work and it did not feel like a hospital because people were not really that ill. It was a happy place, a jolly place and a lot of the time, nurses would come to me for advice or to ask me questions.

All the secretaries used to go out on a bus to visit other hospitals to see how they did things. We went to St James's Hospital in Leeds, High Royds Hospital in Menston and Leeds General Infirmary. Once, they started to talk about getting all the secretaries a uniform like the nurses but there were loads of complaints, so it never happened.

I once took my granddaughter into work when she was a baby.

There was a little shop in the last villa on the drive. It sold things that the residents had made. We often saw residents walking around the grounds. One day, a man came in and sat in the office for a while until someone came to collect him. One of the residents would go around regularly with the newspapers. He also liked to listen to the radio. Another resident was fascinated by cars and would go up to the visitors and ask about their car. One day, a resident got out of the grounds and was knocked over.

At Christmas, we would all go out and we once went to Meanwood Valley Urban Farm.

I left in 1994 but was called back in when the Nurse's Home closed. We moved to an office in the mansion. There was a huge wooden staircase in there and some of the doctors lived in the mansion. I was involved with tidying up and getting rid of stuff.

***

CHRIS GORDON

1980

'I'm quite sure that there were some people there who may have lived longer if they had not been removed."

Chris Gordon's understanding of learning disabilities had started at a young age. It was through his diagnosed sister that Chris came to recognise the care and understanding that these individuals needed.

Though this wasn't his inspiration to move into the field of healthcare, Chris had found himself at Meanwood Park Hospital in 1980 as a care assistant. "I had just turned nineteen and I had been in a job for a few months and had just been made redundant. I had friends who worked at Meanwood Park who were doing their nurse training and mentioned that there were nursing assistant posts going so I applied."

"The grounds were really, really nice. Just walking up the huge, long drive and then having to go into the big mansion it was like, 'I've only come for an interview.' It was just sort of like huge. The hall, or as we called it; The Mansion, that was like the nucleus wasn't it. As far as I know, I believe that was when people first started being admitted to Meanwood, I think they resided within the hall. But yeah, it was really quite impressive, I mean it could have done with a bit of decorating, even in those days, but no it was impressive. You walked in and there was the big stairway and then different sort of corridors off to different admin places and that."

Chris had just passed through the entrance of Meanwood Park Hospital when he had his first interaction with one of the residents. "Strangely enough, on the actual first day I was going into work, I met one of the residents who came over to me and grabbed hold of my hand and walked up the long drive with me. He was living on the villa where I was sent to work. I don't know, I suppose it's quite ironic really because this particular resident was one of the more vulnerable residents who would wander and disappear and if I had not been going there at that time and he had not latched onto me he could have wandered away."

Chris' assigned villa as a nursing assistant was an all-male home in which he remained for six months. "It was fit for purpose but then again [it wasn't.] The sleeping accommodations were just large dormitories, but I wasn't aware of anything else, everywhere was the same at that time. The people that were there, they had adequate food, adequate warmth, clothing; even though the clothing wasn't the best of stuff, but you know their needs were met. So, you may have like 25/26 people living there and, on a shift, you might have three members of staff. In the later years, they started reducing the size of the villas so you might have three staff to seven people which was obviously [more suitable]."

Due to the decreased staff numbers, a lot of the daily routine was structured for staff ease. "It had a bathroom which had, I can't remember if it was two or three baths, but in the same room, side by side. You had like three people, no privacy, three people sitting in the baths like a bit of a conveyor belt like you know. Get them washed, get dressed and down for breakfast. Nobody had any luxuries of thinking 'well, I'd like to sleep in today.' Your shift started at 7:30am so [you took over] the night staff. Many people may be up but if they weren't up by 7:30am it was like, 'this is it now, time to get up.'"

When residents did get up and dressed, many of them were confined to hospital-issued pyjamas which Chris was never too fond of. "They didn't have their own individual pyjamas, they [were] supplied pyjamas [that were] brought in and everyone had them matched up. Hopefully, staff would try and match the colours together but you got some that didn't seem to so you would see two people walking around in like blue trousers and a red top. Everyone had, I believe, a clothing allowance so if you had somebody whose shirt was torn, you could either send it in a repair bag and repair it or if it were too much you'd send it in a condemned bag and then another shirt would be replaced with the person's name stitched into it. Then, they tried to give out these nylon type jumpers which were all the same and were hideous so everybody looked the same and I will hold my hands up and say that we used to get these jumpers and I would personally and with other people, put them under the chair leg and pull them, 'oh dear, that's torn out of recognition' and send it back and ask for something of better value."

As the years progressed, residents were encouraged to have their own nightwear brought in by visiting relatives or, if they were able enough, be encouraged to go shopping to buy their own. "The only [problem] was the central laundry. All of the clothing just got thrown into laundry bags, sent off to the laundry and you may not see that item of clothing again; it may come back again and would fit a toddler or it may fit someone who is 63-stone." Through these unfortunate mishaps, changes were made to introduce individual laundry services on suitable villas.

Despite a lot of the residents being capable of tending to their own hygiene, they didn't have the opportunity to show it. "Lots were independent and to be honest with you, they didn't have the chance to show that. Rather than saying to somebody, 'is there something you could do for yourself?' It would be like, 'right, now it's 7:30am' and there would be a queue waiting for the bathroom. You might have something on a Thursday evening [like cutting] everyone's fingernails and toenails. You had all these regimes put it [place], there was nothing personal in that way. Everyone sort of had bowel records, bath records and that and as much as everyone had a name, within the actual working regime, it was just like a number."

Industrial Therapy continued into the 1980s and so did the tedious tasks. "During my nurse training, we also had to spend an amount of time there. There was one [task] which was like your toilet U-bends and they had to screw these together and pack them in a box and it was like piece work, it was horrible and this particular time, they were all done and somebody who was running the place at the time decided that the staff should unscrew them all and give them back to be redone and I must admit at that time I had to say, 'I'm sorry, but while I'm in here, you're not doing that, that is just so unfair.' There were other things such as packing birthday cards. You had to pack in, I don't know, packs of 50? And again, I was told off really because whilst I was there, I said to the residents 'I'll do them!' And [we] managed to get quite a lot done. So yeah, it was quite exploitative really, some of the things that people had to do. Separating screws and nails and why? Why give someone a bag of mixed [screws]? Why mix them up to have someone take them out?"

Chris did believe that Industrial Therapy was beneficial for the residents, not the tasks that were imposed, but the social side of the therapy. "I think it was beneficial that people could go, they could meet and greet, they could meet friends and it wasn't always the same people from each individual villa. They could make enemies and why not? It's where they could have arguments, they could have chats. I do think that it had a beneficial issue to it but not the actual work that was being done. It would say it was more like a social thing and in some ways, it probably gave someone an incentive to do things or a purpose in some way because you would get, it wasn't much but, you would get an amount of payment from it. The hospital had the resident shop which opened on certain days so they could go and buy sweets. I'm not sure if they sold cigarettes there but I think they did and they could buy the things that they wanted so yeah; it did have its benefits, but it was crap."

Besides the shop, Chris remembered several other patient facilities on-site. "On one of the villas [was] the dentist, not that there were dentists there all the time and not that it was the best of places but they did actually have an operating theatre so if anyone did need any dental care under general anaesthetic it could actually be given there. There was a prefab hut that was the hairdressers. I wouldn't say that you got the option to go in and have any style that you liked, you'd go in and have your hair cut."

Alongside the battle with the general public, inside the hospital there was a driving force to remove the term patient. "When I first started, you still had some of the nursing staff who would wear the nurse's uniform and they would call people patients and we fought really hard to say 'no, we call them residents.' The terminology we have now for where I work is 'clients' which again is wrong because they should really be called 'people', they're people that live there, they've got names."

Alongside the term high-grade and low-grade, Chris also recalled hearing about a third term, babies. "…and the babies which was horrendous. The residents between themselves all sort of like worked from that hierarchy. They would [aim] to be high-grades and they would, to an extent, help with the other people. You then had the people that really, really needed far much more support and although I never heard it from staff members, thank goodness, but I had heard from some of the other residents and they'd say, 'their one of the babies.' Probably people that needed feeding and a lot more support but there was definitely a hierarchy. It was an important hierarchy for the people that lived there."

I'd like to think that the reasoning behind the term 'residents' was done to highlight the fact that the institution was their home and not a hospital. Prior to the community care drive, residents in these institutions were believed to remain permanent fixtures of the place, never moving into the outside world. "I would think that they thought it was home. One of the residents used to say all the time 'oh I'll never get out of here will I?' I don't think they really had any desire or knowledge of what they would have wanted if they got out of there."

Alongside the focus of referring to them as residents, changes were being made to create a more homely environment within the villas. Temporary dividers were being implemented by arranging wardrobes between beds to create individual bed spaces. Towards the end of Meanwood Park Hospital, Villa 14, which was previously closed, reopened as 14 Field View. This was one, if not the main villa, that focused on rehabilitation and independence with the aim to prepare residents for the community. This villa is covered in greater detail further into this book.

Visitation had slightly increased during the 1980s, with family members being more present at the hospital. "There were quite a lot of visitors. When I started it was like Saturdays or Sundays you could have visitors, but the hospital did impose a visitor's regime which again was something that was fought against. You would have two o'clock on a Saturday afternoon, everybody, all the visitors, would start coming in and that was difficult because you were in sort of like the big villas. You had visitors but you didn't have any privacy as everybody sat in the same dining area or same, as we called them, day rooms."

Into the 1980s, the stigma attached to the hospital and to the disability continued to be present within the general public. One popular misconception was the frequent sound of an alarm. "Every Tuesday morning there used to be a fire alarm test. When the fire alarms went off people used to say, "oh I've heard the alarms, someone's escaped". It took a lot of time educating the general public of the area. In relation to the residents, many continued to have no interaction with their family members on the outside. "I always do feel that a lot of people had a lot of guilt. They had them put into Meanwood Park and nothing more to do with them and that unfortunately still prevails. [There are some] still around with us that had been moved to

Meanwood as a toddler and had no family contact ever since."

"There was one resident that I supported and their mother did come and visit them and this particular resident, they had Down's syndrome and apparently, their mam told me many years ago now, apparently when Mum became pregnant again she was told that, "if you do not have your child moved to Meanwood Park, the child you have in there now will be taken away from you as well."

When the opportunity surfaced, Chris applied to the on-site School of Nursing, undertaking two years of training to become a State Enrolled Nurse on Villa 3. "The school of nursing was part of the nurse's home and it was just at the end of the top floor and basically there was a classroom and an office, nothing much more really than that. It had like a big communal lounge area where people could sit and there was a canteen in there and you could go get your lunches if you were lucky enough to have any time to go and upstairs, there were two floors which as far as I know were single rooms where the nurses lived. I went to many Nurse's Home parties which I must admit were quite interesting."

As part of his training, Chris rotated amongst a number of the villas at Meanwood Park Hospital while also having a short, general nursing placement at St James Hospital. "You had to spend a period working in Industrial Therapy and Occupational Therapy and you had to spend time working out in the schools. There was an internal school within Meanwood Park but there were also external schools. I think one of the things that was noted was that at a certain time, I mean I couldn't tell you when, but it was decided that there would be no more children admitted so from a certain time it was just adults only." The internal school that

Chris is referring to is the Department of Education between Villa 10 and 11. "There were only three villas that were classed as children's villas, but I remember, it was based around a big courtyard which was sort of like just classrooms off from there. Eventually, that did close and they moved to just outside the hospital, the school is still there today, Penny Field School."

Standing to the north-east of the original hospital grounds, Penny Field School was opened on the 1st February 1982, replacing the Department of Education at Meanwood Park Hospital.

One aspect of Meanwood Park Hospital that didn't see improvements was the use of antipsychotic medications to neutralise difficult behaviour. "I think that medication, like you say, was used, unfortunately, more [for] control, apart from your anti-epileptic medication which had to be there. But it was the way of the world but in some ways, it was a necessity because you were in a situation where, at the time, you couldn't cope or you couldn't function and you've got other people there that could be hurt or neglected. If you've got some psychiatrist that's going to come in and say, 'oh, I'll increase that or do this' at that time, you wouldn't have thought about questioning that. Therefore, you'd end up with people that were on such large amounts of antipsychotic medications which didn't need to be."

"There was the chief psychiatrist, Dr Spencer, and you'd phone up and say, 'so and so has been such and such.' 'Oh right, I'll come across and we'll increase the Chlorpromazine.' He was nice, a gentle guy really, he would just sort of float onto the villa. You might have been sat in the office and he'd come in and he'd open the filing cabinet, get someone's notes, write something and disappear again but no, he was a nice enough guy."

One medication that was brought up was Chlordiazepoxide. This medication was introduced in the mid-1950s and was primarily used as a sedative. In altered doses, it could also be used to treat anxiety, to control muscle spasms and manage the symptoms of alcohol withdrawal.

"It's difficult because in a lot of ways it was a necessity, an unneeded necessity but because you had three people working [with] so many residents that had challenges, it was [used] as a chemical restraint. We did start getting registrars, so you were getting fresher ideas over the years which was really quite good."

Partnered with this were physical restraints. Chris explained that a few of the villas he worked on did have isolation/side rooms and despite them not being padded, they were used to calm challenging residents. "The unfortunate thing is that nobody, until the latter years, were actually given any training in physical restraint. You would have somebody who would [throw] chairs and wardrobes and it's been a case of [getting] hold of them and if you like, it's awful to say, pin them down. You may have had other people come and help you. I can remember some of the ladies that caused problems and I'm not talking about straightjackets, but they had what we called strong dresses which were dresses made out of like indestructible, well supposedly indestructible, material but it wasn't nice you know." When physical restraints weren't sufficient, Chris confirmed that sedatives were also used.

Eventually, Villa 3 moved towards closure due to structural concerns and Chris was offered numerous villas to relocate to. "We sort of had an option of which areas we may wish to work in and I had never worked with people who had challenging behaviours so I said, 'I'd like to transfer to Villa 12', the male challenging behaviour villa. As soon as I'd asked for it, I thought 'why did I say that?' For the rest of my time within Meanwood Park, I actually worked with people with challenging behaviours."

As a nurse, Chris had some dealings with the on-site mortuary. "[It was a] very strange place [and there was a fridge which had three shelves. We had one of our residents pass away and their relatives wanted to come see them so I just got a phone call to say can I go get this body out for the relatives to see. I did actually ask one of my staff members if they'd come with me and that was quite traumatic really because you opened the fridge and fortunately Ross, at that time, there was only one body in there because they weren't labelled. I pulled the shelf out, thinking like you do when you see on television when the shelf comes out and stays there, it doesn't, it drops; managed to catch it and by which time some porters had come and they sort of then moved this lady out to be able to be seen. The mortuary had some weird things around like jars with brains in other parts like pickled if you like. I think that was from, I wouldn't remember his name but, on Villa 3 there were rooms upstairs which nobody went to because it was so haunted but there was some doctor that used to be there and I think they were like his experiments and things, he'd kept all these things it was very strange. [It] was previously, apparently, used by a former doctor [and] was very much a 'no go area'. Throughout my time working on Villa 3, I was never aware of any of the villa staff venturing into the rooms at the top of the stairs. I did on a couple of occasions go up the stairs on Villa 3 with another member of staff, but nobody would enter the rooms located there."

Amongst staff, Villa 3 had a reputation of being haunted. This may have originated from the war time when it housed an operating theatre. When the war came to an end, the theatre was renovated into the dental suite. "There were strange things, and I can say that I'm quite sure that I saw some things [as well]. There were quite a few of the villas that were haunted but Villa 3 had the reputation for that. Sometimes you'd get a feel but again whether that's because you're young and impressionable. I mean the stairs leading up to where the doctor's things were, I think I went up a couple of times, dared to go up with someone to have a look but I'm sure one time I was walking and there was a figure stood on the stairs but I didn't look twice."

Celebrating birthdays, Christmas and other special occasions was something that Chris was immensely proud about. He saw the opportunity to make residents feel acknowledged and more than just someone locked away in a hospital. "We always used to try and have celebrations and those things. Again, because you've got people living within the settings that there were, things like your birthdays, we'd always go out and buy birthday presents. Christmas' used to be really good for them, we'd try and have good times and in a lot of ways, the staff and the residents all partied together and now, that wouldn't be possible in this day and age but that was a case of staff could actually sit and have a drink with residents. I think a lot of that was staff trying to compensate for the fact that we were working with people who may have not had their own families. My best friend that I worked with, her husband and their friends always came dressed up as Santa and I know it is a bit sort of like, you might think it's like a children's thing but we can all do that can't we? I came to fancy dress parties dressed up as Santa and we used to just, Christmases were lovely you know, a really good time."

As the mid to late-1980s came about, the drive towards community care began to balloon. Despite the emphasis on getting suitable individuals out into community settings, this didn't always work with many returning to the hospital. One of the main criticisms from Chris, and many others who were around during the closure, was the lack of resident knowledge from those in charge of resettlement. "I do honestly believe that initially they got it wrong. If they had input from the staff who were working with these residents, they could have said 'well actually, she can't stand that person, why are you doing this?' Or 'if this person moves they're going to lose so many friendships.' Many of the individuals in Meanwood Park Hospital had friends spanning back decades and when they moved out, they never saw them again. You had people that came, people that needed Meanwood Park, needed that stability. They probably lived there for thirty/forty years or they may have lived there for two years but within two years, you can become dependent on it."

Through a vacancy, Chris transferred to another care provider in 1993 with residents from Meanwood Park Hospital. He later progressed to take on a managerial role, a role where he had the opportunity to make changes in the way people with learning disabilities were cared for. "I suppose from my point of view, I was more in control in as much as 'we've got this smaller environment now, we can support the people to be able to do what they want to do. It may take a long time, but I'd been there (at Meanwood Park

Hospital) for thirteen years and now it's totally different.' So, it's not controlling people's lives but having more control of being able to help them to self-manage their own lives."

Moving out into the community, Chris saw first-hand the struggles that these former residents faced. "They were being given a choice now such as, 'which cereal do you want for breakfast?' Whereas previously it had been 'well this is what has been delivered, this is what you are having.' You could see the difficulty that these people were having."

"We've got people that have far more opportunities. We've got people who have a better social life than I have."

"I thoroughly enjoyed [my time there]. I had some really good times, some bad times and some sad times but I think that from a social point of view, I made many, many friends and I just think that in some ways I hit it at the right time with the push [into the community]. Looking at where we are today, I think sometimes there's far too much over-political correctness. I think that we moved on, we made mistakes, but we've had a chance to reflect on them and we've also made good progress. When I first started there, the first adult villa that I did my nurse training on, there was the Charge Nurse who had been there, a tall chap, older guy, [wore a] white coat and used to walk along while you made the beds. He'd walk round with a stick and measure how far the bed covers were off [the floor] and if it weren't to his liking, he'd rip them off and you'd start again. So, you've got all that, but we really, really, really did push forward and look into the people rather than sort of the structure."

"I suppose it was fit for purpose. It was fit for purpose a lot because a huge amount of people that were there wouldn't have had anywhere else, their families didn't want to know [them]. It was set in lovely grounds, you can't deny that and like I said, a majority of people seemed quite happy there. I think it was progressing, it was quite a nice time for the people that lived there. I'm sure they could have had better, and they do have better now but for the constraints you had, I think we did okay, I think we did a good job. I will always say that I would never knock Meanwood Park Hospital. I think obviously a lot of its structures and things were wrong but it certainly served its purpose and I can't really think of any people that I ever worked with there who were truly unhappy. I think a lot of people might have been like 'this is my lot; I've got to get on with it.' But there were so many people that were so, so happy, such good friendships."

"I think with the way things have progressed; it is important to realise that it's not wrong to do something wrong. It would be wrong if you did it intentionally but if you're putting [ideas] forward and it doesn't work, then it doesn't matter that it didn't work".

"I'm quite sure that there were some people there who may have lived longer if they had not been removed."

***

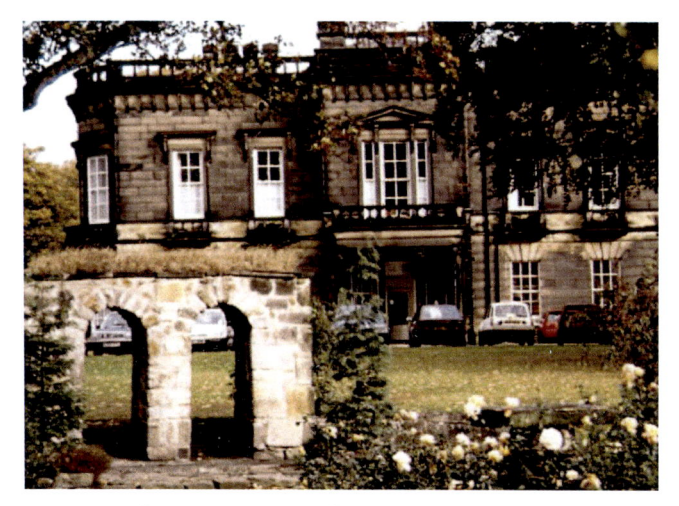

Image from a postcard of Meanwood Park Hospital.

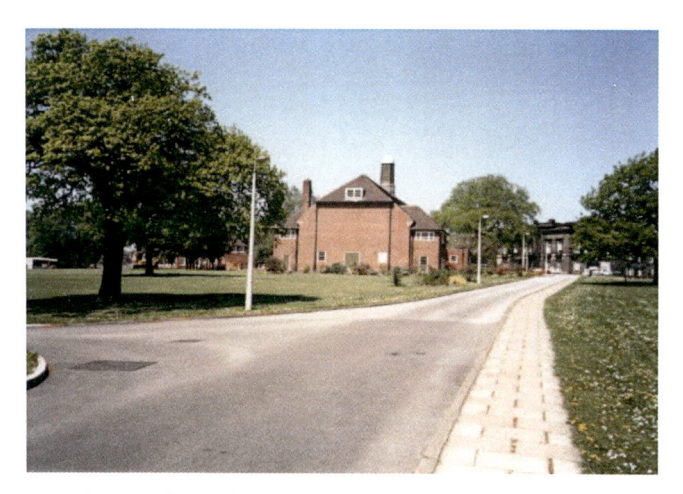

A view up the main drive towards The Mansion – Image by Margaret Hartley.

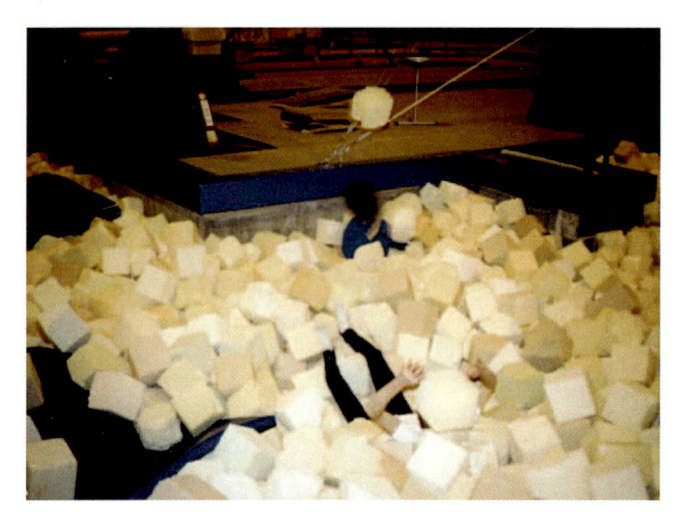

Sunken foam pit for Meanwood Park Hospital residents.

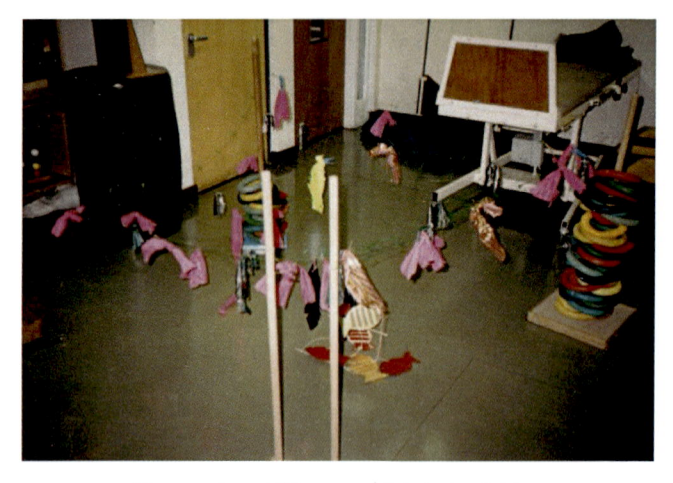

Occupational Therapy/Adult Activities.

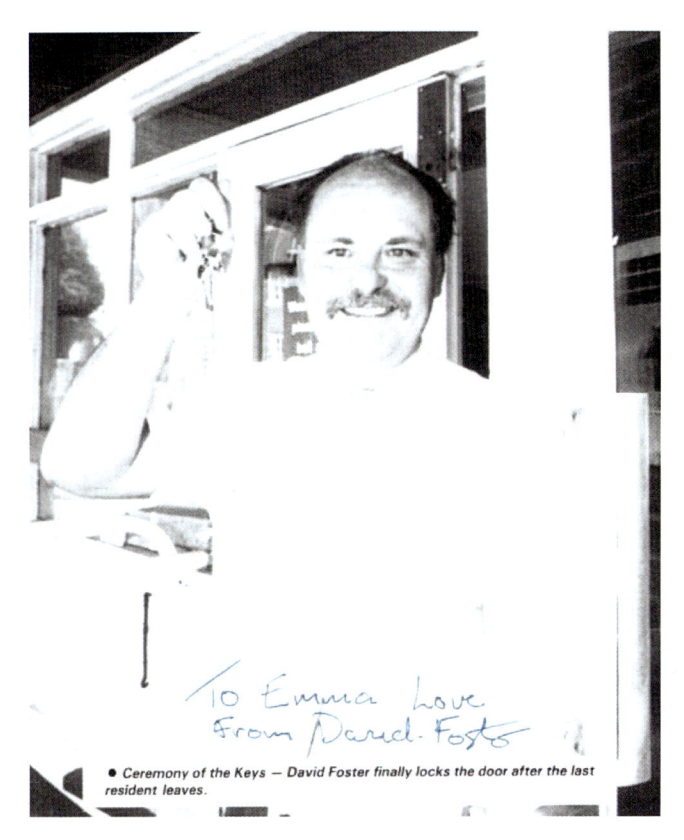

"Ceremony of the Keys – David Foster finally locks the door after the last resident leaves." – Courtesy of *Focus CMH Trust Newsletter July 1997*.

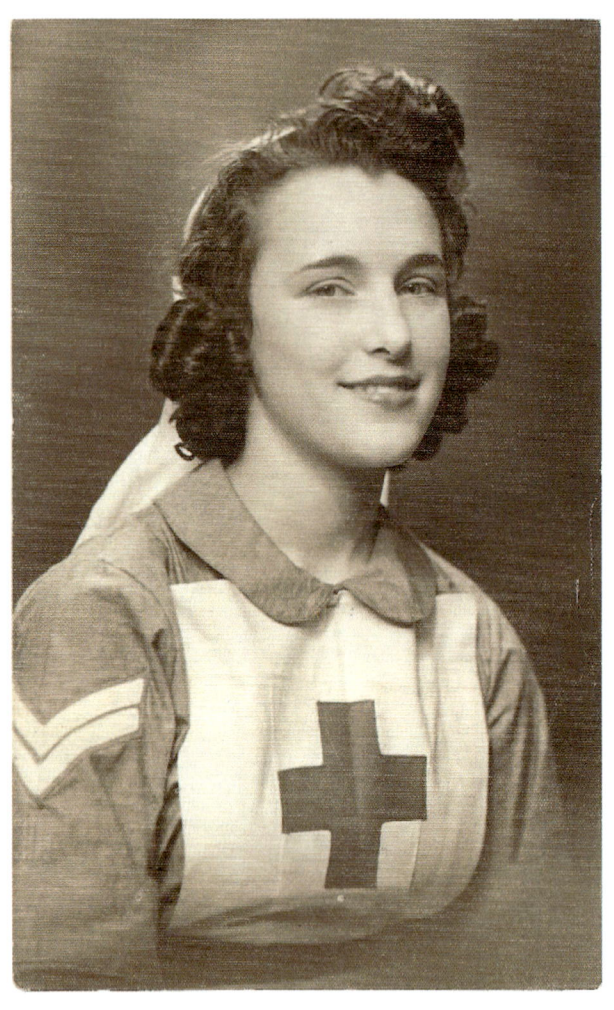

Joan McGrail – Red Cross Nurse during World War II at Meanwood Park Hospital.

VICTORIA WOLFE

1981

"It was a place where a lot of caring went on in an uncaring environment."

During the 1970s, prior to her start at Meanwood Park Hospital, Victoria Wolfe worked as a nursing assistant in numerous institutions for those suffering with a mental illness. Her first facility was Oulton Hall.

In 1925, after being through many uses, Oulton Hall in Leeds became a hospital, providing care for the mentally defective. This remained in use until Monday 4th September 1972 as the push towards community care caused many of the patients to be moved out into residential homes. "For those who still needed hospital facilities it was decided to re-develop the hospital at Fieldhead and the remaining patients were 'evacuated' during 1971 and 1972."[34]

"It (Fieldhead) was supposed to be the most modern in Europe."

Fieldhead Hospital was opened on the 11th July 1972 and, much like Meanwood Park Hospital, made use of a villa system to house its patients. Similar to that of High Royds Hospital, Fieldhead Hospital named each villa after a neighbouring town such as Rothwell Villa and Oulton Villa.

Victoria moved to Fieldhead Hospital with the remaining patients of Oulton Hall and continued there before enrolling at the Wakefield School of Nursing. During her training, Victoria returned to Fieldhead Hospital to undertake multiple placements. She also visited another institution in Wakefield known as Stanley Royd Hospital.

Stanley Royd Hospital was a former psychiatric hospital in Wakefield, opening in 1818 and eventually closing in 1995. The Stephen Beaumont Museum of Mental Health (now known as the Mental Health Museum) was originally housed in the hospital but when it closed, they relocated to Fieldhead Hospital. The museum, which remains there today, includes restraining equipment, a padded cell and former medical equipment.

Four years after qualifying, Victoria transferred to Little Plumstead Hospital in Norfolk in 1980.

This former mental deficiency colony opened in 1930, accommodating over three-hundred patients at its peak. The hospital began a phased closure in the 1990s before closing entirely in the same decade.

In 1981, Victoria returned to Leeds and began working at Meanwood Park Hospital. The transition was effortless as she had worked with similar individuals at Little Plumstead Hospital and despite not knowing much about Meanwood Park Hospital itself, the range of abilities she would encounter were all but familiar.

Victoria explained that Meanwood Park Hospital was more accepted by the local community compared to that of Oulton Hall and Little Plumstead Hospital. "Some patients visited the shops in Meanwood and even though the buildings were old, the atmosphere was better. [At Little Plumstead], everything was on a bigger scale."

Villa 4, a two-storey all-female home, was Victoria's destination however, this was short lived as she left on maternity. "Patients had different diagnoses, ranging from Down's syndrome [and] epilepsy to different physical and mental disabilities." This was one of the villas that partitioned bed spaces to create more privacy. "The large dormitories were sectioned into cubicles to make their own personal space with nice soft furnishings purchased by patients with help of the staff."

On her return to Meanwood Park Hospital, Victoria was relocated to Villa 1. "It was a ground floor building for twenty-three people. It was divided in the middle [and] all but three (residents) were wheelchair users. A [single] member of staff would look after a group of six, supporting them with all aspects of daily living and there was a living room at each side."

With Villa 1 housing those who had more profound physical disabilities, Victoria's time was occupied with medications, bathing, and all other aspects of personal care. "Most needed help with feeding and personal care. I mainly worked nights, so we helped get people up and helped support [them] with meals before leaving the shift."

During the day, residents continued to have access to a variety of therapies. Unfortunately, due to their ability levels, residents from Villa 1 were unlikely to be taken to Industrial Therapy. "A few went out to training centres, some over to Occupational Therapy and some to physiotherapy. We had a music man come sometimes and play the guitar. [Others] went to night school."

In 1996, with the end of Meanwood Park Hospital in sight, Victoria moved into a purpose-built, supported-living bungalow in South Leeds. She accompanied eight of the residents that she cared for in the move to their new home. "The bungalow was semi-detached with four people in each house. I will never forget the day that everyone dressed up and moved into their new home. The move took about a year in all and people were in houses with who they'd lived with and it was a gradual move. The house we moved into had people who had lived together for many years at Meanwood."

"It was an exciting time but for some [residents], [for] staff, a worrying time as they were tupid out with patients going out to the private sector. The people with extra special needs remained in the care of the NHS. The patients were excited as if going on holiday. The working conditions were excellent; the facilities for patients were luxurious and once the move had taken place, relatives were happier. More patients moved into areas local to some family and it was nice how some would drop by for coffee."

Many of the residents who were aware of the closure were known to be excited about their approaching independence while others were not so positive. "One or two found it hard as they couldn't wander around on their own outside, but they soon settled."

Regarding the phased closure, Victoria said that the atmosphere in the final few months of the hospital were dreadful. "Oh, it was awful. I think Villa 2 was the last to go but I can remember one morning, a van turned up and started to strip the roof off Villa 16 and no one thought anything about it as they brought a van identical to the hospital ones. The roofs were slate and worth a bit of money. It was stripped in a couple of hours."

Victoria believed that those who she cared for at Meanwood Park Hospital were capable of being cared for in the community and their stay in the hospital could have been avoided.

"[Meanwood Park Hospital] hid people away, they weren't able to participate in life and develop to their full potential. [It] was frustrating at times, for lots of reasons, but rewarding, making things happen to make the most of people's lives. I look back with affection in that I helped the people we supported on this long journey to where they are living today. It was a place where a lot of caring went on in an uncaring environment."

***

HANNAH HEATON

1983

"It was unheard of to go anywhere else. Your career started at Meanwood, it finished at Meanwood."

Prior to her commencement at Meanwood Park Hospital, Hannah Heaton was employed as an auxiliary at High Royds Hospital, working on a ward that specialised in female dementia. "I didn't really know what the difference was between mental health and learning disabilities at that age, but I could never get into the school. It was always 'apply next year.' So, I applied to go to Meanwood, and I got a place, left High Royds on the Friday and started Meanwood on the Monday."

In April 1983, Hannah began her training to become an Enrolled Nurse at Meanwood Park Hospital. "…you went into the School of Nursing which was on site and you did six weeks in school. You [then] went on to the villas and the villas were all a bit different. They had kids, adults, rehabilitation, physically handicapped and elderly. You did six weeks at St James's Hospital and then six weeks in the school [on-site]."

"The grounds were beautiful because they had gardeners galore. They were lovely to walk around in, they were nice and well kept. I remember it having some swings and there was one patient who used to swing on them forever. There were no tables and chairs outside or nice gazebos, things like that, those things just weren't done there. Villa 1 and 2 were set quite far back and if you did nights it was like you were in the woods."

Today, the training involved in becoming a nurse is demanding and both mentally and physically exhausting. In 1983, that was no different as Hannah's cohort immediately decreased in size with four of the six dropping out.

It is important for students to get experience in as many areas as possible both then and in today's world of nursing. At Meanwood Park Hospital, due to the nature of some residents, numerous villas were unsuitable for students. The villas that Hannah worked on as a student included Villa 9, 13, 1, 2 and 16. "I did what they called 'leisure and recreation'; hated it. Six-week stint and it was supposed to be what they would probably call Occupational Therapy today. You just played games and did those sorts of things and took people out for the day."

Despite singling out Villa 9 as her favourite placement, Hannah did recall two residents that were confined to their rooms during the evening due to their behaviour. "When I look back now, it was bedlam. We had two residents that had to be locked in their bedrooms on a night because of their behaviour and they were then let out on a morning after everybody else had got up and got out. They were sort of allowed on the villa when everybody else had gone or most of the people had gone. When I look back now, it was nothing. One of them used to just go around [making noises] but we had one and they used to just grab somebody's hair if they went past, staff and patients. That's why they weren't allowed." Hannah did remember one of the residents who would proceed to bang their head off the wall at any given chance. "I mean their head; oh, their head was a mess, it was like something out of a horror show. They were virtually bald because they kept pulling their hair out, big scabs, oh its awful when you think about it, scabs all over their head."

Though it is uncommon, from an early age, head banging can be associated with autism and other developmental disorders. At the time, Hannah didn't recall hearing about individual diagnoses. "In learning disabilities, there weren't really a lot of diagnoses, they were just 'born like that' and other services couldn't cope, parents couldn't cope, and they were left on doorsteps. You heard a lot of other tales that there were older people that had actually been little buggers when they were younger, might have stolen a couple of pints of milk from the neighbours and ended up being put away and never got out."

On Villa 10, Hannah's least favourable placement, she described the home as being very sparse. "The bedrooms went off and I think there was a little bedroom where about four of them shared. There were a couple of individual bedrooms and it was just literally, lino floor, single bed, wardrobe, and that was it. The day room was just like a lino floor, one TV; bolted to the wall, two settees and that was it and there was a dining room with just tables and a kitchen; a hatch that food was served through." Those who were housed on Villa 10 were known to have severe behavioural problems. "They used to bang their heads against the wall and there would be a big hole in the wall."

A general day as a student was somewhat repetitive. Mornings would involve waking the residents and getting them ready for breakfast. Unlike today where inpatients have a choice in what meals they have, Hannah explained that residents had zero input on what they wanted. "You didn't really ask, 'do you want this or not?' It was, 'that's your breakfast, eat what you want out of it or don't' kind of thing and most of them did. To be fair, most of the patients ate anything that was put in front of them. I remember once on Villa 13, this sauce came in a big jug and we put it on the meal thinking it was a cheese sauce, turns out it was custard. There were no menus, you got what came on the trolley."

Having an on-site store was greatly beneficial during breakfast and other mealtimes as it allowed staff to retrieve food at short notice. "If you run out of eggs, cereal, sugar, milk, and things like that, you'd do a chitty. Somebody would run up to stores and you'd give it to the man behind the counter and he'd disappear for 10 minutes and he'd go, 'right, I'll get it delivered'. An hour later, a porter would come with it, now you've got to order it a month in advance."

After breakfast, residents who had a reduced level of ability were sent to Adult Activities. With the term low-grades and high-grades continuing to circulate amongst the residents, Hannah explained that the low-grades were the ones who spent their mornings at Adult Activities. "Occupational Therapy was for medium [residents] and then Industrial Therapy was for quite high-grade residents because they used to make little things, do woodwork and they were all on-site." Other than those, connections to outside resources were limited. The ones who couldn't attend any of the therapies would remain on the villa while staff tended to the beds and did laundry. "Very few went to a charity thing like Jewish Welfare, they had a little college out there."

There was one high-grade at the hospital that Hannah remembered fondly. "There was a little old man called

Brian, oh he was ancient, he must have been [in his] late 70s and he was like the high-grade to John, who was the low-grade, and to his dying day, he got him up, dressed and washed."

The Leeds Jewish Welfare Board was established in 1878 and continues to provide a variety of support to the community. "Known as the Board of Guardians the object of the organisation was to provide a broad system of relief to those who needed it and in so doing stop the need for door to door begging and to encourage people to embark on earning an honest livelihood."[35] These Guardians would visit local institutions to check on the welfare of the people under their care.

"Every Thursday, the Rabi used to come round and visit the Jewish residents on each villa, however many there were, I'm not sure how many they were and they seemed to enjoy him coming, they were aware of him coming."

The remaining residents, to Hannah's memory, received little to no visitation but she believed that due to the lack of friends and relatives visiting in the first place, they weren't too affected.

Villa 13 was allocated to Hannah for her short number of night shifts. She would arrive for an 20:00 start and begin organising supper for the residents which would consist of a cup of tea and a biscuit. Villa 13 made use of a lift which allowed those who were less able, the freedom to move around the home. "When the telly finished in those days at about 11:30pm; there was no TV on after that, this is 1983/4, [we] would put as many as we could in the lift, about six of them, go upstairs and put them into bed. We would then go back downstairs, get the next six and put them to bed and it just went on just like that. In those days, it was all dormitories so we would sit from about midnight with a blanket around us because it was freezing, a little night light and you didn't have a phone to play on so you either took a book or what have you and we would sit there all night, just going round with a torch every now and again. As soon as it got to 6am, we would go downstairs, and we would have a cup of tea and then we would be back in the lift to start bringing them all back down."

In relation to nightwear, blue or beige was the colour of choice with nylon being the material. "…they were just pyjamas tops and pyjama bottoms and that was it. They slept in them summer, winter, and autumn. I remember once, after I had qualified, I was working with a woman and we were doing the medications. I said to her 'who is Stephen?' And she went, 'blue pyjamas' and when I went out, they were all in blue pyjamas." The residents that Hannah worked with had little to no interaction with their relatives so the option to wearing their own clothes were extremely limited. "Contact with their families was little until they died, and they would come out of the woodwork because of the money. Some of them people there died with thousands of pounds because they were still getting paid, I don't really understand how but they were still getting their benefits but not spending it."

Those who did receive benefits were often taken on shopping trips. "I remember we used to draw it out, go to the cashier and you could withdraw any amount really you wanted as long as you took receipts back. So like, if there was Fred Blogs, I could go draw out £300 and then I could take him all over town and buy him clothes, trainers and all that and then I could take him for a big swanky meal and then put their receipts in. Then with the clothes, you had to send them up to laundry so they would be named."

"It was a nightmare at Christmas because when it was starting to loom, you'd have maybe £100-£300 depending what they had in the bank and you'd be saying 'right, I'll get him that jumper, I'll get her that radio and I'll get him that mug'. You had to keep all the receipts separate; it was hard work and we'd always buy them a bottle of booze; a sherry or whatever."

"I remember every Christmas on Villa 16, we had a Christmas party and staff went, patients went, relatives went, other villas too and we had every spirit going. It was like a proper party, staff used to get drunk, not the staff that were on duty, if you were on duty you weren't allowed to drink."

Many of the residents who were in Meanwood Park Hospital would tell stories of how they ended up in the hospital. "I remember an old man, Peter Brown, I actually used to bring him home for the weekend and he just used to be what was known as a bit of a tearaway now. He could nick a couple of pints of milk off people's doorsteps, he'd knock on their doors and run away and then he got put in there for like behaviour and never got out."

Residents being taken home with staff for the weekend was a common occurrence, it gave the individual an opportunity to see a new environment while still having that nursing care. The request had to be submitted to those higher than Hannah, most likely the Charge Nurse and psychiatrist. "I used to bring him home, he was hard work now when I look back. I used to bring him home on a Friday night and he would just stay in my house all weekend. I might have taken him for a walk in the wheelchair and he was aware, I used to ask him 'do you want to come to my house?' In fact, there were two residents who used to say, 'is it my turn this weekend Nurse Julie?' I might have had family round and had a bit of a laugh because they were bright enough to fit into that. They knew my family and didn't have kids then. I would take them back Sunday morning/afternoon."

In 1985, Hannah qualified as an Enrolled Nurse and was approached by the Nursing Officer of Villa 16. Hannah, having an interest in elderly care, quickly accepted. "It was different then, that's how you did it. You didn't get interviewed, you just tucked into your role." Towards the end of their training, students were allocated a free placement which allowed them to work on a villa of their choosing.

Villa 16 was a single-storey home with both male and female residents mixing. It was primarily used for wheelchair users, individuals with mobility issues and those with mild learning disabilities. "It was one big, long single-storey building. Some of it was cordoned off as a day room with a TV and then there was another little room that the Charge Nurse used to spend half the afternoon watching the cricket, a few of the patients used to go in there too and watch the telly. Then you would go down and there was a toilet with three sinks and two loos that had doors so you could shut them. There were two bathrooms and we tended to use one for men and one for women. It had three dormitories; women at bottom and then two [for the] men at the other side."

Celebrations for special occasions became more regular towards the mid-1980s, with yearly bonfires being organised by the porters. Hannah's husband, Adam, worked at

Meanwood Park Hospital in the same period as a porter and was regularly involved in organising the bonfire. "Christmas was always lovely. All the villas used to be trimmed up and if you were on duty, staff used to go round in silly hats and to be fair, all the management, as in the Nursing Officer and the big top dog there. Every Christmas Day he would go around all the villas and he'd say hello to all the staff and say hello to all the patients. You don't see them for dust nowadays. It was quite a big thing Christmas and they would get Christmas dinner, turkey and presents." For birthdays, residents would receive a card, balloon and a present and at Easter, they would receive a chocolate egg each.

Alongside these celebrations, residents continued to leave the walls of the hospital for holidays down to the coast. Butlins remained a popular destination and this was one of the locations that Hannah attended. "They were a laugh. I remember one year; we took ten patients; five wheelchair users and five 'walkers' to Butlins. I look back and I don't know how we did it, lifting people on and off the toilet, taking commodes with us and that was a laugh. I remember lifting people onto rides like big wheels, Mexican Hats and Cyclones. Resident holidays were brilliant. We tried to take them away every year and we'd draw their money out and go get them a load of new clothes for their holidays and bits and bats that they might need. Apart from that week away and the odd day out, the trouble with Villa 16 was that a lot of them were in wheelchairs and a lot with zimmer frames so if you only had three staff, you can only physically push three patients unless other people can help."

Adam recalled regular trips to the local pub with a few of the residents and Hannah remembered taking a few to the

Christmas light switch on in Leeds. "There was no real bother. The really violent ones wouldn't have been able to go out anywhere, some were more or less like jolly and happy to be out and a bit loud and boisterous but you trusted yourself to go out with them on your own in those days." If staff had taken residents out for more than four hours, they could claim a meal to the value of five pounds.

Based on Hannah's continued experience of learning disabilities, she explained that today's standards and policies have greatly increased the risk of harm in those individuals. "I think like a lot of things at Meanwood, it was quite staff oriented. Staff had the last word and when I compare challenging behaviour then to now, some staff just had to look at a person who was deciding to pull the curtains down and boot the telly in and they wouldn't do it whereas today, it's 'let them do it, it will calm them down.' In those days, there were consequences for behaviour like that. If they kicked the Christmas tree down, they didn't go somewhere the next day. A lot of the time, people were clever enough to know, they'd get a look from the staff and they didn't do it. In those days there was no need for rapid tranquilisers, there was no need for seclusion, there was no need for restraints, sometimes a look would just do it. I think challenging behaviour has escalated so much and it has gotten more dangerous." Much like today, de-escalation techniques were used that included distracting the resident from the issue. "You'd say 'Mavis, don't do that, you're going to bang your head. Come on let's go watch telly, let's have a cup of tea.' You tried to do that but then when they got so high, you'd go say, 'you know not to do that don't you?' And they'd stop being naughty."

If medication did need to be prescribed, Hannah would speak to Douglas Spencer. "He was lovely, really nice, pleasant and polite. He had a heart of gold and he'd do anything you asked him." With the area of learning disabilities not being a popular area to specialise in during the era of these institutions, Adam explained that the introduction of new psychiatrists was relatively low which resulted in a halt to the standards of resident care. "They were continuing to use old techniques regardless of the improvement in care and science, there was no progressive thought."

Hannah was made to move on from Villa 16 as the home eventually closed. All the residents were moved to the Alexandra Wilson villa which had seized as a children's home. Between the removal of the children and the introduction of Villa 16's residents, the building cared for young adults. "It was not fit for purpose and they went on to AW which was renamed as Beechwood and that became an elderly villa." The children, to Hannah's recollection, had stopped being admitted to the hospital towards the mid-1980s.

Hannah began to hear rumblings of closure towards 1994. "I've worked in this Trust now for nearly forty years, you hear mumblings, mumblings, mumblings. You can hear mumblings for two or three years and then bang, it goes. It happens. A lot of staff had been there since time began; I would still be there now if it hadn't shut. Staff either retired or left in a wooden box basically. It was unheard of to go anywhere else. Your career started at Meanwood, it finished at Meanwood."

As the end of Meanwood Park Hospital approached, staff were interviewed in preparation of moving them into community placements. Residents were none the wiser, with many of them being unaware of their impending removal. Those who were suitable for group homes were separated based on their level of intellectual capacity and physical ability. "You'd have all your wheelchairs in one home and all challenging behaviours in another. I don't think any resident had a say, they were going [to that home] end of."

As the hospital entered its final few days, the quality of care remained despite the steep decrease of resident numbers. The grounds continued to be well maintained, stores and deliveries continued as normal. "I would say it was kept up right to the end."

"When we left Meanwood, we had a choice between Bungalow 5; challenging behaviour/respite or Bungalow 2, which was for those with a profound multiple handicap at Woodland Square at St Mary's Hospital. Even though at that time I was working in challenging behaviour, I chose to go back to physical, what they called then, profound mental handicap."

In 1997, after the doors of Meanwood Park Hospital closed, Hannah continued her career at Woodland Square. She described the setup as being more homely. Residents had their own individual rooms which improved privacy. "There were massive changes from 1997, we got a lot more psychology input and sociology input etc."

Regardless of the improved conditions at Woodland Square, one of the negatives of this move meant that former residents of Meanwood Park Hospital didn't have access to a secure open space. St Mary's Hospital had no tea rooms and the homes in Woodland Square were contained in a small cul-de-sac. In their former home, they had a free reign to travel amongst villas to see friends.

Unlike the lack of advancement in care at Meanwood Park Hospital, Woodland Square saw an influx of Registrars which resulted in fresh ideas in how to care for the residents, including the introduction of Care Plan's and improved activities.

One of Hannah's issues with institutions such as Meanwood Park Hospital was the struggle of catering to everyone with limited resources. "It was environmental issues - somebody wanted the telly on, and somebody didn't and things like that."

Hannah remained at St Mary's Hospital until April 2020, being redeployed due to the COVID-19 pandemic.

"I loved it. I did, I loved it. I've got a lot of memories of patients and staff which I still work with today. I never saw any abuse; all I saw was staff speak highly of patients and do their best in the circumstances. The grounds were well kept and you could have a bit of a laugh in those days, not at their expense but with them. I liked it and I was sorry to see it close, not from a patient's point of view, from a selfish staff point of view."

"I think it was fit for purpose at the time, I think there were a lot of worst places people could have gone. I've never been to any of them but from what I heard; I think there were a lot of worst places people could have gone. They got plenty to eat and drink and people who could make themselves a cup of tea [were promoted to]. Obviously, those that couldn't, you had to get rid of the kettle before they threw it at you. Your Nursing Officer and the so called 'people above you in charge' knew what they were doing, today they haven't a flaming clue. In those days it was a well-oiled machine. The actual buildings themselves were crap and the actual facilities in them were very sparse, very basic but I remember once, when I was on Villa 10 which was for challenging behaviour, we had plastic cups, plastic plates and the telly was chained to the wall. One nurse came in and they said, 'no, no you can't have this, we are having mugs and we are having this, we are going to be normal.' Anyway, when everything got smashed within five minutes, he soon thought 'now I know why they have plastic cups.'"

"They thought it was their home, none of them knew they were getting out. I think they were content with that because they didn't know anything else and I don't think they could have coped anywhere else. It was just sad that there were so many of them in one place, like thirty-odd where now they've gone to [much] smaller, individually supported houses. Staff really tried their best, but we had such limited resources."

***

GEORGE WALKER

1984

"It is much harder to make friends in society than it is with people you live with."

In 1984, George Walker, unemployed at the time, undertook volunteer work at Meanwood Park Hospital through the help of the voluntary services team run by the Leeds City Council. "They said that they had a few things, but there was a place called Meanwood Park Hospital, which I'd never heard of. 'They're looking for people to volunteer to work with people with learning disabilities. Would you fancy doing that?' And I said I would." The only previous experience that George had with people with learning disabilities was through a Christmas party for local children with disabilities whilst still at school.

"I walked up a very long drive one afternoon ... to a big stately building in the middle, and it was quiet, it wasn't scary but it was slightly daunting I think; because of the setup, because of the physical nature of the place and the building. As you went in, I was supposed to go to an upstairs office and there was a big staircase. It was a bit, quite like the Adam's Family house I was thinking at the time, and I can't remember there being any reception. There was a library [in there] and I spent some time there, reading up on a few things. But yes, it looked a bit [different] to the kind of dour brick buildings or the new prefab ones [at the hospital]. This small stately home type thing in the middle is not an unusual model as I've found since then, it happened quite a few times really across the country. People ended up being put behind a big wall on the outside, there wasn't a gate to it, but there was a wall that sort of marked the boundary for the outside world or to the Meanwood world. Not that the Meanwood world was a bad place, that thing about 'was it all bad?' There were bad things but there were some good things. There was a real sense of camaraderie and a sense of safety inside, which you don't get on the outside. Some of the places [today], the service users have less freedom to wander about freely than they used to."

"I met one of the Nursing Officers, militaristic, very nursing way of working. He gave me a short interview, 'yes, I'm sure you'll be fine. I'll introduce you to the Sister.'"

George had exceedingly high praise for the Sister he worked with. "I went in there and she was brilliant. She was one of the most inspiring people that I've ever worked with and she fired my enthusiasm. Initially it was just sitting with people or taking people to say the shop in Meanwood."

"I remember being asked to try and teach somebody to tie their shoelaces. At the time it seemed bizarre because I thought 'can't you just buy some slip-ons', but there was a thought at the end of the tunnel, educate people to be more independent which was an idea that, yeah, a good idea that; this idea of normalisation, trying to get people to be able to slip into society better so they could do things like other people in society, so when they eventually did go live in the community that they could integrate better."

George was rewarded for his enthusiasm as after two weeks, he was offered a Nursing Assistant position at the hospital. "I was offered a job because there was a shortage of staff, even though there was mass unemployment, where there was a shortage of staff in the industry. So, I took the job and did an interview with the same Nursing Officer."

George was allocated to work on Villa 17 which at the time, housed thirty residents with mild or moderate learning disabilities across two floors.

"There was a big central room which was the day room with a fake fireplace, chairs and settees. At the other end there would be a small room, the Quiet Room I think we called it, which perhaps people would use for visiting relatives. Next to that would be the office. Sister spent quite a bit of time [in there], although not as much time as some of the other Sisters or Charge Nurses as the male senior nurses were called, she was much more hands on. At the other side of the day room would be the dining room and the kitchen. There would have been about thirty residents [all male]. I think the youngest would have been maybe late-teens/early-twenties. We had some people in their seventies with mild and moderate learning disabilities and maybe [also] … a physical disability. There wasn't a lift or anything like that, there were steps up to a dormitory for thirty men and they all shared the same bathroom. You would have a bath that is full of water, and you'd have someone getting undressed to get in that water, or someone in that water, and you would change that water [after each use]. So, someone getting undressed, somebody in the bath and somebody getting dry. In the next room, people would be lined up having their teeth cleaned, sometimes with the help of some of the other service users. The more able service users sometimes would help with the care of some of the least able service users."

"Whilst I was there, the role of Villa 17 was to provide an environment that prepared residents for an eventual discharge. A lot of the work we were doing was trying to help people build skills so they could live [more independently]. It was already known that the hospital would close, although it hadn't gone through all the top end procedures, so we wanted people to be able to move out and live [more] independently. During the time I was on that unit, we moved four people into a flat in West Leeds. It was almost like, not a rehabilitation unit in respect, but it would be a unit that helped people learn some self-help skills or shopping, cooking, cleaning, those sorts of things. I loved it."

"[On Villa 17], we were encouraged to have some of the food and to sit with the service users to kind of model how to sit and eat at a table. We were trying to create that feeling of how you would sit together as say, four people and share a meal. Some people found it very difficult, some people would steal other people's food and that kind of stuff because they'd never had that. So, trying to create a learning environment around not rushing your food, all that kind of stuff, cutting [it] into small pieces so you would sit with them and eat and model it while you were cutting the food for some of the people, some of it was liquidised for some people."

Occasionally, staff were moved villas for shifts to cover for shortages of staff elsewhere in the hospital. "I remember the first time I went on Villa 1, this was a villa which housed people with more profound levels of intellectual and physical disabilities – many being in wheelchairs, ... you had two members of staff for eight people with multiple learning disabilities. You would have to get them up, give them a bath, do their teeth if they had teeth, a lot of people had their teeth taken out, give them breakfast, have a coffee and by that point the dinner trolley would come; because that took you about the first half of the shift. It was quite like a conveyor belt of physical care ... and as a male, I often got moved onto Villa 12 which was for adults with severe challenging behaviours; [all male]. I think I was physically scared when I worked there, possibly because I'd heard stuff from the other staff at the time about how difficult it was and how difficult the service users were. Villa

12 was closed down because it was not a nice place. There were too many people in Villa 12 with challenging behaviour, so they split it. If you group too many people together who have got challenging behaviours and triggers, they can trigger each other, so I think that was seen as a sensible move."

What alarmed George the most at Meanwood Park Hospital was the quantity of medications in use. He explained that on Villa 17 the residents were seen as the least difficult with the most moderate or mild levels of learning disability. "...yet the trolley was full of drugs. Mainly, I think there may have been a few barbiturates being used, Largactil rings a bell and you know there were tranquilisers, major tranquilisers." George was unfortunate enough to witness some of the residents display behaviours associated with long-term medication use. "[One resident] had this thing called Tardive Dyskinesia where their tongue would constantly come out of their mouth and it is a known side effect of long-term use of one of those drugs. There was another resident who would kind of go catatonic at times and again, this was because of long term [tranquiliser] use, and really heavy sedation. Previously, they may have had behavioural challenges, but maybe that was a justified challenge to a system that incarcerated them. But because they were directed at staff it would be seen as challenging behaviour, rather than as a legitimate complaint about how they had been kept."

To George's memory, medications were prescribed in large amounts and sometimes given and increased without the psychiatrist interacting with the resident. "I'd like to think that things are moving along but actually, psychiatrists still over-prescribe. [Psychiatrists] don't take kindly to criticism from each other let alone from anybody outside it (psychiatry). They now have a thing called STOMP". "STOMP stands for stopping over medication of people with a learning disability, autism or both with psychotropic medicines."[36.]

"STOMP is a registered campaign setup with the support of the Royal College of Psychiatry to stop them (their own medical/psychiatry colleagues) from systematically over medicating people with learning disabilities and/or autism. Psychotropic medication affects an individual's mental function, behaviour, and experience. Even now in 2020, Public Health England says that every day about 30,000 to 35,000 adults with a learning disability are being prescribed psychotropic medication when they do not have the health conditions that the medicines are licensed for. Children with learning disabilities or autism are also prescribed these same powerful psychotropic drugs 'off licence', and too often."

Diagnoses other than mental handicap was uncommon during George's time at the hospital, with many of the residents receiving this diagnosis without being assessed by a qualified clinician. "There was a resident who was in there who could read and write; they were deaf, but they went in as a teenager because I think their behaviour was a bit, like some teenagers are. But because people couldn't understand what they said, they had no proper diagnosis and once you were in there, you were in. Moral turpitude I suppose would have been the term they would have used."

"Apparently, again I didn't see it, it was via hearsay, that in the psychologists' office there was a cattle prod that had been used, [an] electric cattle prod to give negative reinforcement to some of the service users, to try and extinguish behaviours that were seen as maladaptive as they would say, inappropriate, challenging. I never saw it, but I heard there was one there; in fact, that was from [a] psychologist that was there at the time. It would have been used before the 1980s obviously, they tried to start using more psychological strategies to help people's behaviour, some of it was yeah, very 'do to' rather than 'work with' and today, would lead to a P45, and possibly a jail sentence; but in those days, it was seen as scientific."

For some residents' holidays, George and his group of residents were housed in guest houses or hotels that specialised in providing accommodation for those with learning disabilities. "…in fact, one of the mums came on one of the holidays and we were thinking, 'oh God, can you imagine? We've got to be on our toes all the time, Beryl's mum is coming along.' Well, she had us up playing cards and drinking whiskey and she really had a fantastic time and actually, it was a really enjoyable time, we had a great time, and the residents had a great time. I mean, I did lose someone at Blackpool Pleasure Beach once, which took a good fifteen minutes to find them."

Blackpool Pleasure Beach appeared to be a popular destination and George had many stories to tell. "One time, we took eight service users onto the Pleasure Beach and found the Big Dipper. There were about five of them who were quite able really, so we said, 'do you want to go on the Big Dipper?' And one of them said 'yes' and I knew they were a bit nervous, so I said, 'well I'll go too'. [The rest] stood with the lady who was with me, another Nursing Assistant. So, I sat them together, two there, two there and then I was sitting next to this one, who I think is a bit nervous. We paid our money and the service user got scared and he just dashed off, so as I turned to say 'alright, it's going to be alright' and they'd let this thing, the carriage, go. So, there are four people on there, on their own, and I hadn't checked if they were strapped in or anything; and how long it takes to go round. Of course, they've come back, and they had a fantastic time; and I'm shaking. I think it sometimes shows that we were very protective of people aren't we, and very often they are far more capable if they get the chance."

To George, the public's perception was nothing more than a passing thought. "To be honest, you were often too busy to notice. But I have heard stories from other people, who have heard people say, 'they shouldn't be allowed out'. I recently got told about an incident at the posh Café in Roundhay Park, somebody had asked someone to turn their service user around because they found it 'disgusting' to watch when they were trying to have a meal. Luckily, the staff member told the person to 'fuck off.' So, it is still out there, but I don't remember that much of it to be honest, but I think that's because I wasn't looking for it and I was too busy making sure that everyone was there and engaging with them really."

Visitation for the residents at Meanwood Park weren't always that regular at the time. The stigma in society attached to people with learning disabilities sometimes created a barrier between themselves and their loved ones. Also, distance sometimes played a part: "A lot of people who were in Meanwood Park, their families lived quite a long away-away. [For some], it was a difficult trip and I think some of the older people had no family left. There was certainly a lot more stigma about it, the very fact that it was behind a wall where people were put away, literally."

The terminology used to identify these individuals in Meanwood Park Hospital was continuing in the right direction. "It was clear that they were not seen as patients, there was nothing wrong with people just because they had a learning disability; although they did have a lot of other comorbidities, physical aspects, mental health issues. But just having a learning disability didn't mean you were in a hospital that required being called a patient."

George remained on Villa 17 for over a year before moving onto 14 Field View, which was a unit designed specifically for residents being discharged into the community. "[It was split] into four flats, and we had four people in at a time [in each flat] and we tried to school them up to move into a residential placement in the community."

The aim of 14 Field View was to replicate the residential environment that would be found outside of the hospital, an environment that many of the residents would move into over the coming years. Residents would have their own bed space, or bedroom if available, and would cook and eat together in a communal dining room. "…downstairs they had cordoned off areas with curtains. I think they ran out of money when they were doing it up, so they didn't renovate downstairs into bedrooms. People came through quite quickly. In the end, probably six months I would think their average stay, before a place was identified and they moved on."

Those who were most capable of living outside the hospital were the ones that originally passed through 14 Field View, but more individuals with more complex needs began to be rehabilitated when they realised that they were capable of being more independent if given the support and opportunity. "…we got kind of confident, and we realised that everyone could move out, it didn't matter, they just needed the right placement, and they would be fine."

It became evident that if many of the residents were given time and encouragement, they were able to complete many domestic or living tasks with minimal assistance. "I felt a sense of, when people were given the chance to do things at the right pace, not expecting too much of them, they had much more potential than perhaps was thought beforehand."

One of the most difficult issues with moving residents into a community setting was the obstacle of making new friends. "It is much harder to make friends in society than it is with people you live with, so sometimes that worked and sometimes it didn't. [Residents at Meanwood Park] used to come and visit staff that they knew in different villas and come round for a cup of tea, and they'd do that independently: and where else could you get that? Can you replicate that in the community? No, you can't because you don't know that many people round about the place, and … people are still not that welcoming of people with very clear differences. [Our service users] don't make friends at the club and the pub and the shop perhaps like other people do in society, but they had friendship groups there and sometimes romantic [relationships] which would probably be virtually impossible in community settings."

After six years working as a Nursing Assistant, George decided that he had reached a point where he had done as much as he could in that role to help improve the wellbeing of the residents he cared for.

In his time at Meanwood Park Hospital, George believed that the standards of care had generally improved, with improvements to the physical condition of most of the villas and upgraded staff to resident ratios, such as on 14 Field View. Towards the end of his time at the hospital, patient admissions had dropped radically with people only being admitted as a last resort. "They tried to find other placements for people, but if they couldn't, some people did come in; straight to Field View actually or onto Villa 17 when I was there. But it was a handful of people and it was because it was an emergency admission, there was nowhere else to place them, so they came. Unfortunately, some of those people got stuck in the system."

"I worked through a positive time at Meanwood. I mean if I went as a volunteer and had gone to one of the other villas where people were still sat in rows and rocking like that classic model you know, all dressed in brown, not always wearing their own underwear because it was all put in a big [bag]. If I had been there for a fortnight, I wouldn't have gone back. But I was lucky to get on a villa with a nurse in charge who was clear in what she thought was right, she wasn't hierarchical, she wasn't the old school of 'I tell you everything, you go and do it.' We felt like we were together as a team."

"I was lucky I think, the villas that I worked on were working towards a positive outcome. It wasn't just incarcerating people for their lives, away from society, which was its (the hospital's) initial purpose. I think it had come to a place, I mean society in general had come to a place where they saw that it was morally wrong to separate people because of a learning disability, and they were trying to find, within the NHS it was, a means of getting people integrated into society, not fully but to some degree and it's still an ongoing process. In that kind of sense, it was a positive time in terms of moving people out. There was always still though that feeling that it had been used as a place to put the wrong people … nobody should have been put there, but [some] people got put in because they didn't have a learning disability, they were put in for other reasons. [The residents] on Villa 17 and initially on 14 Field View, should never have been in Meanwood Park Hospital; they would have been able to function quite well in society, given a modicum of support rather than being incarcerated. They were deskilled and became reliant on people and became anxious about society."

"I think one thing about the closure of Meanwood, a lot of the service users, the ones who could articulate a view, said 'this is our home.' Many people had been there for decades, some people had been there sixty-some years and it's the only home they had. The staff would perhaps be the only family they really had, yet some were moved out against their will. Was it the right decision? Probably in the long run, but it impacted on some people in an extremely negative way."

When George left his role as a Nursing Assistant at Meanwood Park Hospital, he went into teaching however, his departure from the hospital was short lived as George returned a few years later to teach some of residents in the hospital's Further Education Unit.

"[We] were using a thing called the Waldon Approach, which was trying to teach, not self-help skills, but trying to teach people cognitive skills that enabled them to develop their general understanding ... we would do matching and sorting skills and movement-based stuff where they would come to us for two hours and we would do one-to-one work. It was called an asocial approach; we sat behind them or stood behind and they engaged with the activity, and if they wanted to engage with us as the only other human being in the room, we would ignore them completely; so we didn't make eye contact. Once we got them sat down, we were trying to focus them on this important activity. Unfortunately, a lot of the service users didn't find that as attractive as trying to engage with you (the teacher), so often there was lack of control, trying to refocus them on this activity that ... in the long run didn't do any good, I didn't think."

George's time teaching at Meanwood Park Hospital was brief as the impending closure of the hospital site forced the educational unit to relocate. "The education aspect was transferred to Leeds City Council and we got a building at Headingley Castle, which was behind The Original Oak, a famous local pub, actually. So, I worked there for a few years."

"With my kind of teaching style, the curriculum changed, and I didn't like this thing they were doing, this asocial approach. I felt it was morally wrong. It treated people as 'other'. I ended up doing an Advanced Diploma in Special Education with the Open University ... I found this thing called Intensive Interaction which was what I ended up doing for twenty years afterwards. Intensive Interaction is a socially interactive approach used to develop improved social outcomes for people with learning disabilities and/or autism. The approach is now widely used by parents, carers and teachers, and focuses on the use of the 'Fundamentals of Communication' i.e. those socially interactive communication abilities that are used prior to the development of speech, these including: sequenced sounds and movements, exchanges of eye contacts, facial expressions and physical contacts."

George went on to work specifically in the field of Intensive Interaction and progressed to work for many years as a Highly Specialized Practitioner and Intensive Interaction Project Leader for the NHS. "I was training people to do Intensive Interaction, and doing research and writing, and doing some hands-on work with more challenging people."

"My role was to try and provide proactive strategies that over time would make their level of challenge reduce naturally, because they would be less triggered, and there would be more interactive relationships with the service staff who supported them ... unfortunately, what [had] happened was ... everything was taken away, all the stimulation that might arouse people was taken away and I went in and said 'let's engage with people, let's sit close to them, let's make eye contact, let's use physical contact' and they looked at me and you could tell that they, some of them, wanted us to fail. Unfortunately for them, we didn't."

***

ADAM HEATON

Personal Account

I was employed at Meanwood Park Hospital as a porter/driver between 1984-87, aged nineteen to twenty-two.

The hospital mortuary was a small brick building on the exit drive out of the grounds. I was involved in the collection of two deceased residents during my time at the hospital. The process involved a metal gurney on wheels with a metal "lid" that was used to transport the deceased from their villa to the mortuary. There were two porters involved to facilitate the transfer of the body, as the sheet wrapped corpse had to be lifted from their bed and on one occasion, carried downstairs. Once in situ and with the cover in place, the trolley was wheeled around the grounds to the mortuary where the body was placed. I cannot recall whether there was any form of refrigerated space, but I do recall it being very cold, gloomy, and foreboding inside the building.

The porters worked a number of defined job roles/shift patterns between 07:00-19:30 on five days over seven rota system. If I remember rightly, there were eight of us in total, varying in age from around twenty up to mid-sixties.

The daily schedule was as follows:

07:00 - Breakfast trolley delivery to each of the villas via two trailers attached to electric floats, later vans. There was always a scramble by the porters for left over sausages, eggs & toast from the kitchens at breakfast time. Milk & bread delivery to each villa via electric milk float. Dirty laundry collection from each villa (first half) via van and delivery to the laundry.

09:00 - Collection of breakfast trolleys. Collection of second half of dirty laundry.

12:00 - Delivery of lunch trolleys to each villa.

13:00 - Collection of lunch trolleys. Delivery of clean laundry to each villa. Delivery of ordered stores supplies to each villa.

The "storeman" seemed, to me, to be around eighty years old and had been there since the dawn of time. On one occasion, I ventured into the loft area of the stores building and came across boxes and boxes of World War II gas masks and other protective equipment, presumably for use in the event of an attack/bombing of the site. There were also supplies of wooden clogs (with hobnail soles) and cotton coveralls that I presume were standard issue for the residents in times gone by.

14:00 - Daily trip out to St James's Hospital incinerator and to refuel vans if required.

A couple of the nursing staff would intercept the porters on the afternoon run at lunchtime with cash and betting slips to place bets at the bookmakers and money to purchase quarter bottles of spirits and cigarettes from the off-license/shops on route.

There was one Nursing Assistant who I will name as he died far too young around ten years ago. Ian Walker was a real character who spent the majority of his shifts studying the racing pages in the Daily Mirror then cadging a lift into Meanwood in order to place his daily bets. My wife, Hannah Heaton, was his lead nurse and spent half her time looking for the absconded Nursing Assistant. He was her brother-in-law, so the frustrations were always taken in good humour. I am sure that any old hospital employees who read the book will remember him with fondness.

16:30 - Delivery of tea trolleys to each villa.

18:00 - Collection of tea trolleys.

Typically, there were four or five residents that would accompany the mealtime delivery drivers to "assist" with getting the trolleys from the trailer into the villas and out again - although only ever one at a time - this caused some degree of consternation on occasion when more than one resident wanted to hitch a ride. They preferred to ride in the milk floats rather than the vans as they were open sided that allowed easy access/egress.

There were Occupational Therapy and Industrial Therapy buildings on site where the residents would attend on a daily basis during the week. The League of Friends ran activities and fundraising events at weekends with an annual fete being held in the summer months. There was also a sweet shop on site where the residents could purchase treats with their earnings.

The hospital was like a self-contained village, with departments for gardening, works & engineering - if anything needed fixing it was done in house.

The residents were, mainly, free to roam the grounds as they desired. None of the residents ever seemed to feel the desire to leave their safe environment or wander off down the road to Meanwood.

To be frank, if a time and motion study had been carried out, the actual amount of work per porter was around one and a half hours per day out of a possible eight. The remainder was spent drinking tea, sleeping, smoking & playing cards or darts with a visit to the Bay Horse or Myrtle for a liquid lunch. There were no qualms about going to the pub at lunchtime in those days.

Weekends were an even more laid-back affair, as the laundry and stores were closed. The only tasks were milk and meal deliveries that everyone on shift mucked in and helped with. The afternoons were spent washing, servicing, repairing our cars and the younger ones used to play football in the courtyard/car park at the rear of the mansion.

All in all, the working life of a porter at Meanwood could be described as comfortable, although after a time it did become rather boring as the tasks, such as they were, were repetitive and fixed.

I believe that after I left, the remainder stayed on until the closure of the hospital.

***

JENNA CRAIG

1986

"Meanwood was of its time. Society had moved on and there was no longer a need for such institutions."

In 1986, Jenna Craig began her journey in Occupational Therapy at Meanwood Park Hospital. The profession had been an interest to Jenna during her time at St Mary's House in Chapel Allerton and off the back of her recent divorce, she believed it was a good opportunity to grasp. "...I didn't want any more time working in an office and saw Occupational Therapy as a career path, but I needed experience to get into University as a mature student."

During Jenna's transition to the hospital, the service she was currently employed at relocated with her and occupied the first building on the drive of Meanwood Park Hospital; the original Nurse's Home. Towards the 1990s, the home was moved parallel to the mansion. The original home was then converted to house a variety of administration.

"On my first day as an OT helper, I turned up at the OT department and was introduced to the staff team and set to work with other members of staff in the department. It was thirty-four years ago so there was no induction process as far as I can remember."

"There were different activities: movement, craft activities, basic cooking, handicrafts, trips out into the community, shopping and I think there was a film show on a Friday afternoon. Various staff ran sessions and I assisted them initially."

During Jenna's time, Occupational Therapy sessions were carried out in the dedicated facility to the north of the grounds. "[They had a] single story office for the manager and secretary, a physiotherapy department, two large halls, several smaller activity rooms and a staff room and there was a kitchen. It was a pretty shabby building, probably passed its sell by date when I was there."

"People were assigned set sessions to attend. These were either morning or afternoon, returning to the villas at lunch time and again in the evening. There was a social element to it as well. We also provided refreshments as well as therapeutic activities, sometimes it was just getting people off the villas for social stimulation. Some people had no verbal communication skills, and some people were very much in their own world and for some people, it was hard to discern how much they were getting out of the activities. Some people you could visibly see they were appreciating the activities. For others, the signs were often hard to distinguish and needed staff that worked with them on a regular basis to interpret their reactions."

In 1987, a Technical Instructor role came available which Jenna was successfully accepted for. Her new position placed her in the Adult Activities department, the area where those with more profound learning disabilities spent their time. Coming from a similar environment, Jenna was able to use her experience to help further improve resident' lives. Working within a smaller team allowed Jenna to establish one-to-one sessions. "[This gave me] an ability to be more creative with activities and an opportunity to take individuals out into the community as we had access to the minibus one day a week and we could also use public transport."

Group outings had seen a dramatic reduction in numbers with an improved staff to resident ratio. Rather than large groups leaving the hospital at once, smaller groups were now being prioritised. Local trips were taken for example to Piece Hall in Halifax, Roundhay Park, Temple Newsam and the dry ski-slope in Harrogate. The former ski slope was believed to have been located on the Great Yorkshire Showground. The slope closed in early-2000.

Many of the residents that came to see Jenna had a range of physical, intellectual, and mental abilities. Self-harm did occur on occasions amongst some of the residents. "Some people exhibited self-injurious behaviour [such as] head banging, and violent outbursts could occur usually due to frustration and/or an inability to communicate their needs. All fell under the umbrella of learning disabilities, some were autistic, some had severe communication problems which may have explained their challenging behaviour." Despite these incidents of self-harm, medication was never an intervention used by the team in Adult Activities. "We would try to position ourselves to cushion them and to reduce the likelihood of injury. Try to calmly talk them down, try distraction techniques."

"One example I remember was a young resident who seemed bent on smashing their head against windows when they were distressed. Another resident, it seemed like they appeared to have no pain threshold at all and would bang their head on anyone or anything. They wore a protective helmet most of the time to try to reduce the impact. We tended to shield other people in the group from danger keeping the distressed person at a distance rather than isolating them or restraining them."

In 1989, Jenna left Meanwood Park Hospital to train as a qualified Occupational Therapist. "I trained in Newcastle at Northumberland University. There were only a few universities that trained OTs at that time. As a mature student, I had to demonstrate that I had studied and experienced OT practice. I had undertaken an OU (Open University) course in Special Educational Needs prior to this. On my OT course, I had three clinical placements a year, all in a variety of settings. Mental health (hospital ward), drug addiction, older people's services, learning disabilities at Prudhoe Hospital in the North East and general rehab; both in hospital and in the community."

Prudhoe Hospital was also an institution for those with learning disabilities. It opened in August 1914 as Prudhoe Hall Colony with the initial aim to house children only. In 1930 the colony changed hands and "plans were made to increase the accommodation for up to 700 inmates."[37] With this increased capacity, the colony prepared plans to create small villages for men, women, and children. "…many of the projected buildings were never constructed, at least in the form originally envisioned."[38]

After completion of her university course, Jenna returned to Meanwood Park Hospital and was offered a time-limited contract which she completed successfully. During her short return, Meanwood Park Hospital was undergoing some much-needed changes. Daily Living Assessments were introduced which allowed relevant staff to review the daily needs of residents to determine if they needed any additional support while continuing to promote independence. "At that time, the predominant philosophy was one of social [role] valorisation in that all people needed support in order to fulfil their roles and were given a greater degree of choice that they had previously been used to." I remember working with a resident who had cerebral palsy and could not use a self-propelling wheelchair. I got a representative from a supplier out to assess her for an electric wheelchair and spent many hours teaching her to use it. This required cooperation with the physio department and numerous adaptations to the control system. She was incredibly happy, and it gave her a degree of independence and freedom."

"I worked with residents with coordination problems to improve their eating and drinking skills by provision of adaptive cutlery and changing the environment. This involved observing the person eating and drinking and establishing what the problem was. This could involve postural adjustments, seating and adapted implements and giving advice to the staff so they could assist. I also assisted the physiotherapists running rebound therapy sessions on the trampolines which were based in the old day service building, a full sized, normal trampoline. When they moved to St Mary's Hospital, they used a sunken trampoline. There were various benefits, cardio-vascular activity, improved coordination, relaxation for people who had a lot of spasm and a sense of achievement and fun and enjoyment."

After her exit, Jenna applied for the Harrogate Hospital Rotation. "I worked for six months on the rotation and then saw a post for a Senior 2 Occupational Therapist based at Fieldhead Hospital in Wakefield in 1994. I applied and joined the OT and Physio Team in Wakefield providing day service for people at the Hospital. I returned to Meanwood in 1995 for a Senior 2 post."

Jenna returned to Meanwood Park Hospital as a Senior Occupational Therapist and instantaneously recognised that the hospital was pushing towards community-based care. "Very much had changed. The therapy teams were now based in the now vacant Villa 6. The day services no longer involved direct OT input. Some of the Villas had closed and the focus was on the closure of the hospital and the resettling of the clients with new providers in the community. Some of the people with more challenging behaviours and mental health problems were to remain under the aegis of the Trust based at St Mary's Hospital."

"By that time, most of my time was spent assessing and assisting the move into the community. This entailed visiting various properties and making sure that the environment was suitable for the needs of the clients that were being proposed to move there. This could involve assessing for overhead hoists, wet floor showers, mobility rails, ramped surfaces, specialist seating, appropriate beds and adapted kitchens if required. We also advised on colour coding to assist people with sight impairment. Colour coding involved using different colours to differentiate doors, floor surfaces, lighting to improve contrast for people who had some but limited vision."

A year before the closure, Jeanna left Meanwood Park Hospital for the final time, undertaking an Independent Practitioner role in the community. "I worked as part of a multidisciplinary team catering for the needs of learning disabled people living in the community, some of whom had always lived in the community and some who had recently moved out of an institution in the vicinity. Some lived with their families and some lived in supported accommodation. It was a more flexible environment in which to operate and it involved being out in the community rather than a hospital or institutional setting."

Jenna recalled that closure had been spoken about during her first stint in the 1980s, but nothing had finalised. "There was an awareness that this would inevitably occur as all large institutions were having to prepare for closure and move into the community."

"It needed to close, and the majority of people now have a better quality of life. However, a section of the Meanwood population were very happy wandering the grounds in safety during the day, visiting other villas and departments and friends in the grounds. I imagine they would have found the limitations of movement in the community a bit daunting. Meanwood was of its time. Society had moved on and there was no longer a need for such institutions. Institutional behaviour still existed in some areas where staff had worked there a long time. If I correctly recall, some very able residents had already been moved out into the community before I started working there."

"My time working at Meanwood Park Hospital taught me a lot about people; it was a valuable experience and contributed to my career. In a later stage of my life it helped me cope with my stepson who has learning disabilities and lives in supported living."

***

TERRY CRAIG

1987

"The Philosophy of moving into the community was fast becoming the way forward."

Jenna's husband, Terry Craig, also worked at Meanwood Hospital during the same period and held the role of Superintendent Physiotherapist. Terry had previously gained experience at an inclusive learning centre in West Leeds.

As a Superintendent Physiotherapist, Terry would be at the front line of resident care. "I was a front-line manager who managed the physiotherapy services for the hospital, Penny Field School, and the day services in the wider city. As a front-line manager, I spent a considerable amount of my time treating patients alongside attending meetings. I was also responsible for initiating a safer moving and handling programme for Leeds Eastern Health Authority."

Terry wasn't solely based at Meanwood Park Hospital in 1987, his presence was also required at Penny Field School. "I managed both sites and had staff that covered both sites, but I was predominantly based in the hospital. The department also covered the learning disability service for adults throughout the city mainly in the city-wide training centres."

At Penny Field School, Terry used a variety of methods and techniques to assess the children's ability levels. "[We used] physical measures to realise their ability potential and prevent their physical state deteriorating which can happen if there is not an intervention to prevent it. For instance, postural management helps to improve the ability to eat. We also did mobility training and hydrotherapy. They were children with serious intellectual and physical problems. The children in Penny Field School lived at home with their families. The connection with the school was that in the past it had taken in children from the hospital. As there were no longer children under the age of sixteen in the hospital, this did not occur anymore."

"I can remember a child whose impairments were the result of a road traffic accident and after many years of treatment, they managed to drive themselves around in an electric wheelchair. I can remember another young child with Athetoid Cerebral Palsy who we spent a long time teaching how to feed themselves."

During the late 1980s, Terry witnessed the change in the public's perception of those with learning disabilities. Despite this positive awareness focusing on children rather than adults, it was a positive step forward. "…it was gradually becoming more positive however, the acceptance of adults with learning disabilities took longer to improve than that of children with similar issues."

Within Meanwood Park Hospital itself, Terry realised the lack of staff resources available to maintain a basic level of mobility for some of the residents. "I realised this was not due to any lack of care. [There were] not enough staff available to do things other than basic nursing/caring tasks. I needed more staff and there needed to be an increase in the number of people in day services in order to get residents out of the villas to do more stimulating activities, both physically and intellectually."

As a Superintendent, Terry had the ability to make improvements and through the assistance of the day services, he implemented posture training with the staff. Terry also liaised with the villas to ensure staff were "…[taking] a more active role in maintaining the existing mobility of residents."

"[There was] a man in his thirties with a mild hemiplegia, epilepsy and a learning disability who had once been able to walk but was now spending most of his time sitting down and not moving. With some encouragement from me and some of the staff we managed to get him back on his feet."

Alongside the required improvements that Terry implemented, he also believed that the atmosphere on some of the villas also needed development. "Some had a very pleasant family atmosphere and some veered towards the more institutional approach. "The villas that had a more positive atmosphere were staffed by younger staff whereas the ones with more institutional aspects were usually staffed with people who had been working in the system for a long time."

Terry was very much involved with Rebound Therapy which he believed was greatly beneficial for the residents. "[We had] a resident with Athetoid Cerebral Palsy who once on the trampoline would wriggle, jiggle and giggle. They thoroughly enjoyed the freedom of movement and being out of their wheelchair. If you spent most of your day in a seated position, then to stretch out on your back and be able to move freely in any direction you wanted without assistance had to be a pleasant and beneficial experience."

Another type of therapy that was provided was Hydrotherapy. For Hydrotherapy, residents were taken across to Penny Field School "[The] aim of hydrotherapy is to move in a non-weight bearing environment. The warm water reduces spasticity, encourages full joint movements, reduces pain and is enjoyable. It kept them flexible, helping to reduce the rate of their contractures worsening. It was also a relaxing and enjoyable activity. Some of the more able residents could propel themselves on their backs almost independently which was a great achievement for them."

The physiotherapy department also provided specialist seating, wheelchairs, splints, and protective headgear. "We also supplied orthopaedic footwear to help correct faulty gaits that many of the residents had."

"I always found a way of communicating with the residents even if some of them did not appear to have obvious communication skills. The nature of my work meant that I had physical contact with them which usually seemed to be appreciated as so many of them had little physical contact other than daily living procedures. Some of the most enjoyable times were spent on the trampoline which was the most conducive environment for building up a therapeutic rapport. Children from Penny Field School also visited to use the trampoline and it was very satisfying to hear the laughter that ensued with them and their staff during the sessions."

Terry remained at the hospital until its closure. "People moved out in stages and in a fairly orderly manner until the last couple of months when the developers were keen to move in and the last few villas moved very quickly. It did get quieter but by this time a lot of our work was being done in the community, so we spent less and less time on site. There were mixed feelings around the site as some of the staff who had been there a long time were very apprehensive, not only for the welfare of the residents but also themselves. [They] were being [moved] to new providers and were worried about their future. I was very positive about the closure bearing in mind that I have a son with learning disabilities and would have not wished him to have been living in a hospital environment."

The physiotherapy department was relocated to St Mary's Hospital and Terry continued to provide a service for those who had resided in Meanwood Park Hospital and adults with learning disabilities in the wider community. As the final days grew to a close, those who had challenging behaviours were allocated a place at St Mary's Hospital while the remaining residents were being placed in suitable accommodation throughout the city. The day services also moved to St Mary's Hospital and the former residents were brought in to benefit from the therapeutic services provided by the unit - "…activities were similar to the ones at Meanwood, including rebound therapy and a much larger hydrotherapy pool."

"The closure was always on the cards from the moment I arrived in 1987. The reason behind it was that it was no longer considered a suitable environment for these people as the philosophy of moving into the community was fast becoming the way forward. There was also a financial incentive in order that to help fund community care, the sale of the land was necessary."

"Some people should not have been there in the first place and those that were there were not realising their potential. It was time to close the place down and probably should have been done a lot earlier. It catered for the people who were there as best it could with the staff resources available and to its credit, had improved massively in recent history. There was no doubt it was an institution, if a rather benign one. The majority of the staff meant well, but society had moved on and it needed to close."

***

ROSIE HOPE

1988

"There were buildings next to each other that housed a few inmates like little families."

Despite originally housing a dental suite in Villa 3, the hospital made use of the community dental team to provide oral care to the residents of Meanwood Park Hospital. In 1988, Rosie Hope was a member of the community team that attended the hospital. Besides her visits to Meanwood Park Hospital, Rosie also cared for other vulnerable individuals such as the homeless and young offenders.

"From my memory, the main house looked lovely, but the buildings looked a bit like a concentration camp, but my memory could be playing tricks. I think it was a layout side by side. There were buildings next to each other that housed a few inmates like little families. Some were trying to get back into the community. They used to go out all day and come back at night much to the horror of the community as they often found one in their house. I was told that the surrounding houses weren't happy as they couldn't do anything about them wandering."

Rosie's visits to the hospital were usually on a weekly basis but was often called out when needed.

Minor procedures such as dental hygiene and dentures were tended to in the resident's communal room. For the more invasive procedures, residents were escorted to a suitable dentist in the community. "It would be a big job getting them sedated if necessary. With special needs and domiciliary visits, it was mainly NHS dentists who dealt with them. Private dentists did see some or would refer them to the dental hospital if they were too difficult. Usually the ones we saw didn't have a dentist." With the community teams only carrying out minor acts of care and the fact that there was the drive towards community care, it leads me to believe that the dental suite was no longer needed.

"[I] never saw it but it was probably antiquated by then. Only at High Royds Hospital did I see a dental suite."

"We had to take what equipment we needed as we had to be mobile to go to different blocks. The minor services included dental hygiene and maybe taking impressions to make dentures. Dental hygiene at a sink and temporary filling if toothache; whatever we were called out to do." The use of a non-sterile area was intriguing but for Rosie, this was a common occurrence. "[It was a] different world to some degree. We worked in whatever area we could to get the job done but we did wear gloves."

Being exposed to the living arrangements of the residents, Rosie was content with the standard appearance. "We didn't go into their bedrooms, but the communal area and dining/living was pretty standard. They looked after themselves a lot, trying to get back into the community. They had like a house master to help them and often guards if they became violent or unpredictable."

"I remember we were asked to see two residents, so we went in the afternoon. We were told they wouldn't be back until 6pm so had to wait. The organiser warned us that one had carried out a sexual assault and the other had caused harm to one of their parents. In those days, I wore miniskirts so I was a bit worried. Anyway, the first one came in and stared at me accompanied by a guard. The second one came in and sat down. The first one needed some impressions, so I started to do it, but he started struggling so I held his arms down, I think we were on the floor by then. Then, a cup came whizzing past my head and smashed on the wall caused by the other resident. The guard took them out and they were gone for a bit and then they came back. By then, we had finished the first one. Second one looked sheepish and said they were sorry then added, 'they hit me.' I remember saying, 'well you shouldn't throw cups at people.' [It was] a bit scary."

"Another occasion we went but couldn't do anything as across the grass was the main house with the big staircase and there had been a serious patient incident."

"[The grounds were] beautiful from what I remember, lots of grass around and flower beds. It was well run and a calming place. It was good to have small communities in the villas and it was homely. The residents I saw were being let back into community gradually, so some were going back home each night and learning to look after themselves. It was therapeutic and calming for them."

***

LEANNE FIRTH

1996

"Seeing the villas cognitively was heart-breaking to me as the reality was that it was very institutionalised."

In 1996, Meanwood Park Hospital had a limited number of months remaining but despite this, Leanne Firth was employed as a Support Worker within the Day Services unit of the hospital. Leanne had taken an opposite approach to many of those in this book, beginning in a community placement at the age of eighteen before moving into an institution at the age of twenty-five.

Despite the decrease in staff and residents, Leanne and many others in similar positions were brought into Meanwood Park Hospital to continue providing care to its remaining few. "The day service took on staff if a vacancy came up and as far as I am aware, the villas were the same."

"I was interested in psychology from a young age and I've always had a great passion for people with learning disabilities. I loved to enable people to reach their full potential. Day Services offered me the chance to do this and I also fancied a change from working shifts and sleep-ins."

Meanwood Park Hospital had been a fixture in Leanne's life from a young age. "I grew up near Meanwood Park, so I knew of its existence. As a young child you could often hear sirens going off at the hospital. We often thought that this was an alarm to alert that someone had escaped but it was only in the later years that I found out it was just the hospital alarms being tested. I remember growing up in Meanwood and attending the annual fairs that would be held within the grounds or watching staff go past my house as they were making their way to and from the hospital. When I started as a Support Worker in the community, training events would also be held within the hospital grounds. So really the hospital was in my awareness from the age of five years old. Subconsciously, as a child, it felt like a sense of normal. I remember having an interest, a kind of empathy when seeing a person with a physical or learning disability. The grounds were beautiful, and the trees were incredible, greenery in abundance. I always remember the villas as looking a little imposing but as an adult, seeing the villas cognitively was heart-breaking to me as the reality was that it was very institutionalised."

During this period of uncertainty, Leanne praised the efforts of those she worked with at the Day Services. The staff continued to create an atmosphere of positivity and focused on the residents in their care rather than the impending closure. "The staff at the Day Service were amazing, full of energy, compassion and commitment for everyone that used the service: progressively thinking, inclusive and had the common ethos that everyone had the right for autonomy. The service is still in existence today. It's now called Ventures and it's based at St Mary's Hospital."

The aim of the Day Service was to provide residents with the tools to live independent lives where possible. Activities were structured to replicate daily tasks such as cooking lessons, shopping, and general hygiene. "It was a full-on experience that's for sure. The air was full of change and this was a difficult time for some people after many years of institutionalisation. Often when community homes were opened, staff who knew their residents well would support the transition and go into community housing to try and reduce people's anxiety. Obviously, people felt afraid and nervous of what was to come. For some, it was difficult as Meanwood Park was a relative haven and if they wanted to nimble to the café run by a group of volunteers, or just potter around the grounds, they could. There were big changes ahead and many had to learn to be safe in the community."

A typical day for Leanne would begin by collecting the relevant residents from their villas. "We'd ring the doorbell and wait; when the person was ready, we'd walk on to the next villa. By the time we'd got back to the Day Service, we'd have a trail of people behind us." Once back at the unit, Leanne and the staff would commence an array of activities such as music therapy, hydrotherapy, physical exercises, and daily living tasks such as cooking. "We also offered Rebound Therapy. Many of us were trained to become Rebound Therapy Coaches so we would work very closely with the physiotherapists, making specific plans for people to use the trampoline to enhance/maintain their physical wellbeing."

"The villas were crowded, and people still had to share rooms in some circumstances. Access to kitchens were non-existent and meals were taken from villa to villa, akin to a meals-on-wheels or hospital style delivery. On some villas it was noisy, limited personal space available and no real stimulation offered. It often felt stifling and conveyor belt-like. Getting people up dressed, fed, medicated. It felt oppressive; lots of institutionalised behaviours were expressed by the residents. Independence, autonomy and choice a person had was very minimal."

Leanne encountered a variety of characters during her short time at Meanwood Park Hospital. One resident in particular had been a permanent fixture of the institution for many years with their family unaware of where they were. "…they used to potter around the grounds, calling out their own name as this was the only word they could say. I never heard them utter another word. They used their name to express their emotions phonetically. If they were angry, they'd say their name angrily. If they were stressed, their name would become high pitched and if they were happy, their voice would sound content. They had no other verbal communication. They also walked with a limp; they were a mystery. It turned out that as a young child, they were playing in the street and had been knocked over. They were taken to hospital and then transferred straight to Meanwood Park Hospital without any attempt to find their family. When I worked at Meanwood they must've been around fifty or so and only a few years before had their family been reunited with them. They had been looking for them all their life and had never given up. They were basically kidnapped and confined due to their learning disability."

Leanne also brought up the terminology of high-grades and low-grades which by that point, appeared to be nothing other than history.

Eventually, Meanwood Park Hospital did close and Leanne was relocated to a residential setting. "The hospital got quieter and quieter, becoming a ghost town where the past met the present in an eerie grey silence. I have been privileged enough to see psychological and behavioural changes from people who have transitioned from the institutionalised environment to a place of freedom, choice, independence and autonomy."

"I was gutted about the green space being destroyed. I was concerned for the people who may have found the change too difficult to cope with. Many of the residents were losing contact with each other and their home that they had been used to. Unfortunately, a lot of the people appeared to be used to loss and frequent changes of staff or they didn't have the capacity to express how they were feeling. No one should have been there at all but sadly, as I said before, many were scared, anxious and apprehensive to change due to being institutionalised. Every time I drive past the wall, I remember an individual telling me they were forced to build the bloody thing. It closed too late and was not fit for purpose as it was historically in situ to pay homage to a different mind-set of an antiqued era. However, I was elated that people had the chance to be free from institutionalised environments. It was lovely to see many people move into their own homes, to have their own rooms and lots of space. Over the years watching people adapt, change, and grow in confidence, eventually functioning to their full potential, has been a total honour and at times humbling. Even though many were only able to have informed choices there was hope for their future, a new existence, a new beginning."

***

SUMMARY

Twenty-three years ago, Meanwood Park Hospital, an institution that evidently struggled due to lack of adequate resources, ceased its services and became an important fragment in the history of learning disabilities.

When deinstitutionalisation began in the 1950s, it initially aimed to remove individuals from long-stay inpatient services and integrate them back into their community to become functioning members of society. It was Enoch Powell's 'water tower' speech in 1961 that marked the turning point for institutionalised care. Although this was primarily aimed at psychiatric hospitals, it also addressed the historic hospital services in the country.

"There they stand, isolated, majestic, imperious, brooded over by the gigantic water-tower and chimney combined, rising unmistakable and daunting out of the countryside – the asylums which our forefathers built with such immense solidity to express the notions of their day. Do not for a moment underestimate their powers of resistance to our assault."[40]

A volume of these plans did not take into consideration that many of these patients had spent numerous decades inside these establishments and simply moving them into a community home would not be an uncomplicated transition. This is evidential at Meanwood Park Hospital where many former residents returned due to their inability to integrate into their newfound independence. Their self-contained community was stripped away, their haven amongst the walls had been demolished and their ability to freely move was now restricted. Although there were many misconceptions of the hospital, such as the weekly fire alarm, the residents were shielded from a world where they were inevitably not welcome.

To say that today's society is accepting of those with learning disabilities would be inaccurate, many of those diagnosed continue to be at the forefront of discrimination. It is the lack of understanding and false assumptions from members of the public that continue to further decrease any opportunities available to these individuals.

Although standards of care and choice were little, several members of staff created environments of inclusion, care and understanding. Birthdays were not ignored and special occasions such as Christmas were enhanced to show the residents that although they were segregated from their relatives, they had a family within the hospital.

Meanwood Park Hospital was an institution of its time. It was constructed with the aim to hide people from society who were deemed unfit. "It became the dumping ground for society's rejects. That's not saying anything about the people who were put there, that's saying something about society."[41]

***

LIBBY HAYS

2020

"They are more involved in decisions as much as they can be compared to before."

I had the pleasure of growing up with Libby Hays from an exceedingly early age and to be able to interview her for this book felt more than appropriate.

Today, Libby Hays is a Deputy Manager within a Specialized Supported Living Service based in Leeds which cares for those with learning disabilities.

Within her service is sixteen group homes with three-quarters of them supporting those with profound learning disabilities while the other quarter is for those with challenging mental health needs. "Profound, we class as full-time wheelchair users without any challenging behaviours. If they had challenging behaviour, then they would be better placed in a challenging behaviour house."

It is important to note early that the individuals in Libby's care are referred to as tenants and not clients or residents. "We call them tenants or service users because it is their home. They have always been tenants to us, we are in their house, we work in their house."

There is a variety of diagnoses amongst the tenants in her care with a majority of them having cerebral palsy. One individual does a nervous system disorder that causes physical and learning disabilities while a second has mental health problems. Only two out of eight tenants in one of the homes can communicate, the others have limited communication. "…you wouldn't understand them unless you knew what they were saying. If you knew them, you would understand but otherwise you wouldn't." Staff consistency is important when creating a rapport with tenants and the staff turnover in Libby's service is exceptionally low. "…staff don't change that often. [An] apprentice joined in late-2019 but before that, the last person that came in was about three years ago, so we don't have a vast turnover of staff."

Unlike in the previous days, the training available to staff in this field is extensive and within Libby's service, all members of staff are Makaton trained. Unlike British Sign Language, Makaton makes use of signs and symbols in conjunction with speech at all times. "…you only sign every other word in the sentence whereas in sign language, you just seem to sign everything, and it can be more confusing for someone with limited communication. Sign language is harder to learn whereas Makaton, you only learn certain words. So, if you're going to say, 'do you want to go for a bath?' you could just say and sign 'bath?' and they would know what you mean. It is simpler."

Many of the tenants in Libby's care came from home while three of them came from Meanwood Park Hospital. Those coming from home are required to go through numerous assessment stages to ensure there is an available residence. "They would go to their social worker and then it would go to a panel to see if they've got a room available. Let's say there are six people in Leeds that need a room, it would then go to the panel and they would see out of them six which one is more suitable for that house and whose needs can be staffed and then they just get picked."

The three former residents of Meanwood Park Hospital have limited communication and Libby believed that their stay in that institution further decreased their already reduced physical and intellectual ability. "I suppose the younger you are introduced to independence, the easier it is to learn compared to someone coming to us now and having to be taught it."

One member of Libby's staff had previously worked at Meanwood Park Hospital and fifteen years later when she transitioned into the group homes, there was one former resident already housed in the group home that she previously cared for.

Independence is highly promoted in Libby's homes and adaptations are made where possible to facilitate this. "They have been deemed unsafe to use knives and kitchen equipment/utensils but with assistance it tends to be fine if you don't leave them with a knife and walk off. They can sort of mix pans and if they are baking, they can crack eggs, it will go everywhere but you just tidy it up."

During the day, many of the tenants will leave their homes for day centres while others rely on outside services to come to them. "…we've got three of them that have outreach support teams that come in for a few hours a day, a few times a week and then a few have a social group which is specifically for adults with learning disabilities. Sometimes the groups go to like White Rose for a coffee."

The day centres incorporate a lot of stimulating and useful activities into the tenants' daily lives. Passive movements, groups activities and weekly discos just to name a few. "One of them that goes has got full capacity, you can have a full conversation with them, he is just a wheelchair user. They enjoy going. They always come home happy [and] have regular reviews with the centre's key workers."

Other than general outings, tenants are usually flown abroad once a year with an additional UK holiday also provided. Unlike the early days of Meanwood Park Hospital where group holidays were done in large numbers, today's holidays are usually done in pairs. "They usually don't go away with more than two. So, if one tenant likes to walk for miles yet another tenant would just lay on a sunbed and they are happy doing that, we wouldn't put them on a holiday abroad together. There are two tenants that are mobile, and they have been going away together for years and that is because they both enjoy walking. There are three members of staff so they don't have to stay together for the whole holiday they can go off on their own. It's two staff to one tenant but if two tenants are going then we will take three staff because the other one can then float between."

Unfortunately, a small minority of the general public continue to look down on those with learning disabilities. "I still think people stare and I think when they go to appointments, sometimes the doctor or the dentist or whoever, will talk to you and not them. I suppose for a stranger in White Rose Shopping Centre, it's their ignorance rather than anything else. When they go into hospital, we stay 24/7 and offer all required assistance, feeding and personal care etc. We still need to be able to say what's recently happened, but I don't think there is enough training as such in learning disabilities. I don't think hospitals are down with positioning or moving and handling either, they just sort of pull them up the bed and stick a pillow under them but they wouldn't understand if someone has a complex body shape to fill the gap in and with pressure sores, they just tap a bit of cream on and move them around. Our guys have sleep systems, and all the staff are posture management trained to aid positioning, I don't think hospitals are down with it."

Amongst the numerous rehabilitation services that are available to the tenants, Hydrotherapy remains a positive choice. "Me and four other members of staff out of sixteen are trained to do Hydrotherapy which means we don't have to do it with a Physiotherapist. [It is carried out at] Armley or Halt Park Leisure Centre. The physiotherapist will complete the training with the staff and create the tenant a programme to use while in the pool which contains the correct stretches to do. The allocated time is between twenty/thirty minutes that you're allowed in the pool due to the heat. Once the exercises are done, if there's any time left over, we just turn it into an opportunity for sensory time. Swaying and splashing or depending on the programme weight bearing which for someone in a wheelchair full time makes all the difference."

Medications are still commonly used in the field, but many are tailored to reduce muscle rigidity and manage pain levels. "The most common is Baclofen, a muscle relaxant. They're all so tense, contracted and then we've got Pregabalin and Carbamazepine. "

Baclofen is a muscle relaxant and an antispasmodic agent. It is most commonly used to treat muscle symptoms caused by multiple sclerosis and spinal cord disorders. Pregabalin is used to treat epilepsy while Carbamazepine is an anticonvulsant.

Unfortunately, residents are unable to self-manage their medications, but efforts are made to include them during medication time by explaining what medication they are being given and its uses. "…we pop it out and we say, 'you've got two in a meds pot' and then give them it. We've got others that take it with food and if you were to give it, you just have to say, 'you've got a yogurt with this tablet on top' and we've got one that's got a peg feed so you're just saying it as you're putting it through the tube."

Methods of physical restraints are to be avoided unless there is a severe risk of harm. Modern behavioural management training looks at identifying the individuals triggers so interventions can be made as soon as possible. If de-escalation techniques are unsuccessful then sedatives can be used. Despite one tenant being prescribed a regular dose of antipsychotics; lorazepam is also administered during psychotic episodes. "The lorazepam is given in small doses. They will have half a tablet every time and if it's not working and we need to up it, we have to ring the doctors before we give it rather than just give it straight off and explain why we've given it and what we've tried to do before. If we were to give him anymore, we'd have to ring them again."

Out of the tenants in her care, she does believe that two of them could be suited to an assisted living environment rather than supported living. "One of them always talks about moving on, they always say, 'I'm going to move out in 2020' but I think it would be hard finding that level of support they require to move out because they can't cook, they can't do their own medications so they would need some sort of input."

Despite living in a community home, Libby believes that many of her tenants are institutionalised, especially those who came from Meanwood Park Hospital. "…you would put their drink down and you're not going to take it away but they will drink it straight away and if you put a packet of crisps down, they will [instantaneously] eat the crisps because they think you're going to take it."

"I think because of COVID-19, it's proved how, I know you shouldn't say it, but it proves how used to a routine they are, getting up, centre on a Tuesday, coming home and having their tea because at so-and-so time, they are wandering the room. I think they are used to routine and I know for a fact that part of having a learning disability is that you do need a routine, for autism you do need a set routine of what's happening."

Four of Libby's homes make use of a sensory room which is designed to "develop a person's sense, usually through special lighting, music and objects."[39] It is commonly used for children who have limited communication skills.

Despite efforts to make the house as non-clinical as possible, it is important that tenants are aware that it is a healthcare setting and certain items need to remain there such as staff rotas and medical notes. "Some tenants could see certain rooms in their house as more office-like as they contain locked cupboards with files in. But as much as it is their house, it's also a workplace so daily notes and MAR (Medicine Administration Record) Charts need filing and there is a picture rota for tenants to see what staff are on shift in the coming days so there must be a happy medium of understanding."

As a Deputy Manager, Libby has regular interactions with Woodland Square at St Mary's Hospital. There is no permanent residency available here, only a respite service for those with profound and multiple learning disabilities as well as those with challenging behaviour. "[It is] mainly used for manager's work - office days, completing paperwork, staff meetings, team training and supervisions/appraisals." One of the rooms at Woodland Square is commonly used for person-centred reviews and needs assessments. "…we would meet with their family or any profession that wants to come and then usually, before COVID-19, it was in an environment where they'd want to go. The tenant will mainly pick a place - the pub or at home with a tea party. I suppose they are more involved in decisions, as much as they can be, compared to before where they would get told what was happening. [They have] tenant meetings to discuss any changes that are needed around the house [and a] PCR (Personal Centred Review) which is done yearly then reviewed throughout the year. If they don't have capacity, then best interest forms are always done. If you were going to redecorate a bedroom or book a holiday, you don't just book Lanzarote because you want to go, you sit down with all the pictures and say, 'last year you went there, this year do you want to go there, there or there.'"

"I think we still do have old school staff in the way that when a new piece of equipment comes in, 'that's not going to work and that's never going to work' but you don't know until you try and times have changed and it's tough shit, you've got to move with the times."

***

MORE FROM THE AUTHOR

High Royds Hospital: An Insight into 'Insanity'
Available now on Amazon in both paperback and Kindle.

High Royds Hospital, a former psychiatric hospital south of the village of Menston in West Yorkshire.

It is evidential that High Royds Hospital provided sub-par treatment for the mentally ill although this level of care was not consistent throughout the hospital's function. Despite inadequate resources, numerous staff created environments of inclusion, promoting the importance of independence, and celebrating birthdays and other special occasions. *High Royds Hospital: An Insight into 'Insanity'* offers a window into a world that many of us misunderstood.

"I never really got over the fact that justice wasn't served." – Elsie Lam

"One lady, Betty, I will always remember Betty, she used to say, 'when are we going to dance?' And I would say, 'when we get this lot to bed!'" – Cora Rowntree

Also available is the short continuation, *High Royds Hospital: 'Madness' in the Memoirs*. Available on Kindle only.

Continue reading for a preview of *High Royds Hospital: An Insight into 'Insanity'*.

CORA ROWNTREE

1974

Cora Rowntree fulfilled many roles during her working years within inpatient psychiatric services, at both High Royds and beyond. Her extensive recollections of her time at Menston's asylum makes for a fascinating read.

It was 1974 when Cora's journey at High Royds Hospital began. In the beginning, she received on-site training to become a Clinical Support Worker, or better known then as a Care Assistant.

Prior to her adventure in psychiatric healthcare, Cora worked as a Silver Service Waitress.

However, Cora admitted that she always had the intention to train as a nurse, originally wanting to nurse the poverty-stricken children in Africa.

Lindley Ward was Cora's destination on her first day at the hospital, which she defined as the geriatric ward for women. Originally, the block where this ward was located, alongside Rigton, was the male chronic block. Based on this development, I am unsure when the switch was made from male to female inhabitants. Cora admitted to having feelings of unease on her first day but countered them with enjoyment. She explained that morning shifts would begin at 7am, running until 2pm, where the afternoon staff would intervene and take over. Lindley is where she first encountered the male Charge Nurse for the ward, who she went on to praise.

When asked if she remembered her first day, Cora replied with "vividly." It had begun with the Charge Nurse asking Cora to help assist one of the nurses with the tea round. Cora witnessed large flasks being filled with hot water and then filled with both milk and sugar. This prompted her to ask the question "what if they don't take sugar?" "Oh yes, they do. Most of them do. You don't have to worry about that." The nurse had replied. Cora admitted that this particular moment had stuck with her ever since.

Much like in today's hospitals, the routines are mirrored day after day and this was no different in High Royds. Cora's morning began by first waking up the patients, assisting them out of bed and helping with a bedside wash. Once a week, patients could find themselves having a bath in one of the three tubs that the ward had to offer. These baths were positioned at the centre of the bathroom and isolated from one another by curtains for privacy. Staff recorded bathing times to ensure everyone's hygiene was maintained. If patients had incontinence issues then additional baths were given. Following this, patients were helped into the wards dining area and served breakfast. With Lindley being a ward for the elderly, a majority of the patients were brought in via a wheelchair. Food, which Cora described as "wonderful," was wheeled in by local porters. I asked if Lindley had a dedicated room for feasting or if it was carried out in a multi-purpose room in which Cora agreed with the latter. Amongst the collection of patients, a nurse was assigned to a table to help feed those who needed assistance. Cora went on to explain that these allocated nurses were very attentive to the other patients, engaging in conversations, ensuring that everyone was included.

Following breakfast, patients were directed towards the lounge where they resided for the remainder of the morning, undertaking a handful of activities until lunch. The lounge, as described by Cora, housed a standard television, a radio and a collection of books and magazines. As the majority of patients had mobility issues, there weren't many intense activities planned during the times between meals, with many patients enjoying the little things such as the radio.

While patients were occupied, the remainder of the staff would head back into the dining room and clean up. I asked if patients were made to assist with the cleaning duties, but Cora confirmed they were not. She said that some patients would return and assist in ways they thought were beneficial but that usually resulted in them picking up loose crockery just to place back down moments later. Staff allowed patients to assist as it gave them a sense of purpose.

The day would continue much like it began, with patients heading off for their next meal before returning to the confines of the lounge.

Alongside general hygiene assistance, Cora and other Healthcare Assistants were allowed to carry out the changing of medical dressings. Cora remembered one patient who had acquired a serious pressure ulcer to the base of her spine.

Pressure ulcers, or sores, occur when a patient remains in the same position for a prolonged period of time. The most common areas for these sores to develop are on the areas of the skin where the bone is close to the surface. This includes the heels, spine, elbows, and bottom.

The continuous pressure on Cora's patient's spine had caused a Stage 4 Pressure Ulcer. This is where the skin has broken down to an extent where the base of her spine was present through a large hole. When tending to this sore, Cora remembered having to wear two face masks. One to protect herself from the open wound, and the second, doused in perfume to mask the smell of the rotting flesh. One of the remedies that Cora carried out included stuffing the wound with bandages soaked in olive oil. When questioned about this, Cora said "Olive oil feeds the flesh, so it helps it to heal. So, we were using that obviously, but she was in so much pain and discomfort." Following this, the patient would be turned onto her side to relieve the pressure, alternating between each side as early as every thirty minutes. Following this, Cora took it upon herself to speak to one of the ward's doctors, which was in fact her first time interacting with one, asking them "why do we let people suffer like this." Looking at the wound, Cora said she knew that it wasn't going to heal. "Her spine started to break down and we had to massage it and when we turned her, we would massage her and everything." Patients' dressings would be changed at minimum, once a day.

To continue reading this interview and many others, please purchase High Royds Hospital: An Insight into 'Insanity'. Available now in paperback and Kindle from Amazon.

NUMBERED CITATIONS

1-2   Atherton, H. 2005. *Unit 2 – A brief history of learning disability.* [online]

         http://www.healthcareimprovementscotland.org/his/idoc.ashx?docid=4e7e450c-1113-4104-8fe2-d6103970a7b5&version=-1

3   Archives Hub. no date. *Legal papers relating to the Denison family.* [online]

         https://archiveshub.jisc.ac.uk/search/archives/a33fedb3-e82d-38cb-b05c-3c7e7db7f1c9

4   Bhimani, N. 2020. *Some historical sources on intelligence testing.* [online]

         https://blogs.ucl.ac.uk/special-collections/tag/history-of-education/

5   Wellcome Trust. 2020. *The Eugenics Society archive.* [online]

         https://wellcomelibrary.org/collections/digital-collections/makers-of-modern-genetics/digitised-archives/eugenics-society/

6   Aanmoen, O. 2019. *The Princess who was gassed by the Nazis.* [online]

         https://royalcentral.co.uk/features/the-princess-who-was-gassed-by-the-nazis-126641/

7-10   Spencer, D. (1989) 'Sketches from the history of psychiatry', *Psychiatric Bulletin,* 1989, pp. 629-631.

11   Langdon Museum of Learning Disability. no date. *Social History or Learning Disability.* [online]

         https://cutt.ly/ugOI8Cn

12-13   Guggenbühl. (1849) 'Dr Guggenbühl's Hospital for Cretins', *Boston Medical Journal,* 1849, pp. 20-22.

14   Bénédict de Saussure, H. (1796) *Voyage Dans Les Alpes*. (n.p.).

https://www.nejm.org/doi/pdf/10.1056/NEJM184902070400105

15   Guggenbühl. (1849) 'Dr Guggenbühl's Hospital for Cretins', *Boston Medical Journal*, 1849, pp. 20-22.

16   Camphill Scotland. no date. *The Camphill Movement*. [online]

https://www.camphillscotland.org.uk/the-camphill-movement/

17   NHS. 2013. *Pennine Camphill Community*. [online]

https://www.nhs.uk/Services/careproviders/Overview/DefaultView.aspx?id=71287

18   Jack Tizard School. no date. *Who Was Jack Tizard?* [online]

https://www.jacktizard.lbhf.sch.uk/about-jack-tizard-school/who-was-jack-tizard

19   WalesOnline. 2013. *Why the Ely inquiry changed healthcare forever*. [online]

https://www.walesonline.co.uk/news/health/ely-inquiry-changed-healthcare-forever-2041200

20   Socialist Health Association. no date. *Report on Ely Hospital*. [online]

https://cutt.ly/vgPOqF0

21   Writing Services. no date. *Theory of Normalisation Drugs*. [online]

https://customwritings.co/theory-of-normalisation-drugs/

22   Department of Health. 2001. *Valuing People*. [online]

https://assets.publishing.service.gov.uk/government/uploads/system/uploads/attachment_data/file/250877/5086.pdf

23	Prabhala, A. 2007. *Mental Retardation Is No More.* [online]	
	http://sath.org/page/Mental_Retardation_Is_No_More151New_Name_Is_Intellectual_and_Developmental_Disabilities/10130/741/	
24	Open Forum Events Ltd. no date. *Learning Disabilities and Autism.* [online]	
	https://www.eventbrite.co.uk/e/learning-disabilities-and-autism-equality-and-empowerment-registration-71631133649	
25	Silver, L. 2014. *Is a Learning Disability Considered a Mental Illness?* [online]	
	https://ldaamerica.org/is-a-learning-disability-considered-a-mental-illness/	
26	Mencap. 2016. *What's the difference between a learning disability and a mental health problem?* [online]	
	https://www.mencap.org.uk/blog/whats-difference-between-learning-disability-and-mental-health-problem	
27	Wessels, D. 2017. *What is lanugo and what causes this hair to grow?* [online]	
	https://www.medicalnewstoday.com/articles/320220	
28-29	NHS. 2020. *Hydrocephalus.* [online]	
	https://www.nhs.uk/conditions/Hydrocephalus/	
30	GraduateWay. no date. *History of Occupational Therapy.* [online]	
	https://cutt.ly/RgPODsN	
31	The Memories Group (1996) *Memories of Meanwood* (n.p.).	
32	WebMD. no date. *What is Microcephaly?* [online]	
	https://www.webmd.com/parenting/baby/what-is-microcephaly#1	

33   Ethical Care. no date. *Our History and Background.* [online]

https://cutt.ly/4gPP3jo

34   New Woodlesford. no date. *Mental Hospital.* [online]

https://newwoodlesford.xyz/oulton-hall/mental-hospital/

35   LJWB. no date. *Our History.* [online]

https://ljwb.co.uk/about-ljwb-2/

36   NHS. no date. *Stopping over medication of people with a learning disability, autism or both (STOMP).* [online]

https://www.england.nhs.uk/learning-disabilities/improving-health/stomp/

37-38   The Workhouse. no date. *Prudhoe Hall Colony, Northumberland.* [online]

https://cutt.ly/ogPAt2u

39   Sensory Room. no date. *What is a Sensory Room?* [online]

https://sensoryroom.weebly.com/what-is-a-sensory-room.html

40   The Health Foundation. no date. *Enoch Powell's 'water tower# speech.* [online]

https://navigator.health.org.uk/theme/enoch-powells-water-tower-speech

41   George Walker Interview

NOTES

Durham Mining Museum. no date. *Allerton Main Collieries.* [online]

http://www.dmm.org.uk/colliery/a204.htm

Leodis. no date. *Meanwood Hall, Drawing.* [online]

    http://www.leodis.net/display.aspx?resourceIdentifier=200576_53115481

28DaysLater. 2019. *Meanwood Park Hospital Mansion – Leeds.* [online]

    https://www.28dayslater.co.uk/threads/meanwood-park-hospital-mansion-leeds-january-2019.116281/

Lincs to the Past. no date. *Portrait of Sir Henry Hickman Bacon in the Upper Great Chamber.* [online]

    https://www.lincstothepast.com/Untitled/945497.record?ImageId=23830&pt=S

BBC. 2009. *Restoration Drama.* [online]

    http://www.bbc.co.uk/leeds/content/articles/2009/07/31/places_roundhay_park_mansion_reopening_feature.shtml

History Collections. 2016. *Inclusivity.* [online]

    https://historycollections.blogs.sas.ac.uk/2016/03/03/inclusivity-a-selection-of-materials-from-the-special-collections-on-education-for-children-with-learning-difficulties-2/

ReduceTheBurden. 2009. *Compulsory Sterilization.* [online]

    http://reducetheburden.org/compulsory-sterilization/

Cygnet. no date. *About Cygnet Health Care.* [online]

    https://www.cygnethealth.co.uk/about/about-cygnet-health-care/

Historic England. 2015. *Crooked Acres Hospital.* [online]

    https://www.pastscape.org.uk/hob.aspx?hob_id=1067944

Secret Leeds. 2007. *Oldest Roads.* [online]

    https://www.secretleeds.com/viewtopic.php?t=70

Ancestry. 2003. *Lees of Saddleworth*. [online]

    https://www.ancestry.co.uk/boards/surnames.lees/262/mb.ashx

Historic England. no date. *Lodge to Meanwood Hall*. [online]

    https://historicengland.org.uk/listing/the-list-entry/1375475

Pearson, A. 2019. *Eugenics: Adam Pearson on science's greatest scandal*. [online]

    https://www.bfi.org.uk/news-opinion/news-bfi/features/adam-pearson-eugenics-science-greatest-scandal

Moyle, G. 2010. *The History of Cell Barnes Hospital*. [online]

    https://www.stalbansoutofsightoutofmind.org.uk/content/place/cell-barnes/the-history-of-cell-barnes-hospital

The British Newspaper Archive. no date. *Yorkshire Evening Post*. [online]

    https://www.britishnewspaperarchive.co.uk/search/results/1942-06-24?NewspaperTitle=Yorkshire%2BEvening%2BPost&IssueId=BL%2F0000273%2F19420624%2F&County=Yorkshire%2C%20England

NCBI. 1969. *Industrial Therapy in Mental Hospitals*. [online]

    https://www.ncbi.nlm.nih.gov/pmc/articles/PMC1982065/?page=1

Hirst, R., Leber, K., Brady, H. and Imbus, C. no date. *History of Mental Institutions*. [online]

    http://psychologyshistory.umwblogs.org/evolution-of-institutions

Séguin, E. (n.p.). *Idiocy: And its Treatment by the Physiological Method*. (n.p.).

    http://th-hoffmann.eu/archiv/seguin/seguin.1907.pdf

The National Archives. no date. *The Royal Earlswood Hospital, Formerly the Earlswood Asylum, Redhill, Records.* [online]

    https://discovery.nationalarchives.gov.uk/details/r/ed87972d-14f1-4b0c-ab59-d72bcdbee573

(n.p.). no date. *Lost Hospitals of London.* [online]

    http://www.ezitis.myzen.co.uk/magdalen.html

Langdon Museum of Learning Disability. no date. *Earlswood Asylum.* [online]

    https://langdondownmuseum.org.uk/research/u3a-research/2014-long-stay-institutions-for-people-with-learning-disabilities/earlswood/

Disability History Museum. no date. *Private Institution for the Education of Feeble-Minded Youth.* [online]

    https://www.disabilitymuseum.org/dhm/lib/detail.html?id=1707&page=2

Britannica. no date. *Francis Galton.* [online]

    https://www.britannica.com/biography/Francis-Galton

NHS. 2013. *A Disability History Timeline.* [online]

    https://www.merseycare.nhs.uk/media/1749/disabiliyt-timeline-2013.pdf

Ruskin College Oxford. no date. *Judy Fryd.* [online]

    https://www.ruskin.ac.uk/story/judy-fryd/

The Health Foundation. 1971. *'Better services for the mentally handicapped' white paper.* [online]

    https://navigator.health.org.uk/content/better-services-mentally-handicapped-white-paper-was-published-department-health-june-1971

People's Collection Wales. no date. *Ely Hospital: Hidden Now Heard.* [online]

https://www.peoplescollection.wales/collections/579951

UK Essays. 2018. *Theory of Normalisation of Drugs.* [online]

https://www.ukessays.com/essays/criminology/theory-normalisation-drugs-8646.php

Mencap. no date. *NHS England to close England's last long-stay institution for people with a learning disability.* [online]

https://www.mencap.org.uk/press-release/nhs-england-close-englands-last-long-stay-institution-people-learning-disability

NHS England. 2017. *Redesign of learning disability services across the North West.* [online]

https://www.england.nhs.uk/wp-content/uploads/2017/03/nhs-consultation-proposals-redesign-ld-services-across-north-west.pdf

Lancashire Telegraph. 2018. *Union Bosses: Calderstones Hospital closure date 'unachievable'.* [online]

https://www.lancashiretelegraph.co.uk/news/16169761.union-bosses-calderstones-hospital-closure-date-unachievable/

County Asylums. no date. *Calderstones.* [online]

https://www.countyasylums.co.uk/calderstones-clitheroe/

Atherton, H. 2003. *Unit 3 – A brief history of learning disabilities.* [online]

https://lx.iriss.org.uk/sites/default/files/resources/NES_Unit 3.pdf

University of York. 2015. *Claypenny Hospital.* [online]

https://borthcat.york.ac.uk/index.php/claypenny-hospital

Crofton, I. (2015) *History without the Boring Bits.* (n.p.).

Hogenboom, M. (2001) *Living with Genetic Syndromes Associated with Intellectual Disability.* (n.p.).

Thackray Museum of Medicine. no date. *History.* [online]

https://thackraymuseum.co.uk/about-us/history/

The Workhouse. no date. *Beverley, East Riding of Yorkshire.* [online]

http://www.workhouses.org.uk/Beverley/

Osburn, J. and Caruso, G. (2011) 'Some Effects of the Transition from Normalization to Social Role Valorization', *Guest Column,* 2011, pp. 47-57.

Physiopedia. no date. *Rebound Therapy.* [online]

https://cutt.ly/EgPDZGO

Learning Disability Today. no date. *Assessment and Treatment Units.* [online]

https://www.learningdisabilitytoday.co.uk/assessment-and-treatment-units/

Drugs.com. 2019. *Chlordiazepoxide.* [online]

https://www.drugs.com/cdi/chlordiazepoxide.html

Oulton Hall Hotel. no date. *The History of Oulton Hall Hotel.* [online]

https://www.oultonhallhotel.co.uk/media/1242/the-history-of-oulton-hall-a5-landscape.pdf

Dutta, S. 2019. *History of Tuberculosis.* [online]

https://cutt.ly/lgPD5xh

Culture Grid. no date. *Killingbeck Smallpox Hospital.* [online]

http://www.culturegrid.org.uk/search/2156807.html

DerbyshireLive. 2018. *Derbyshire miners angry over planned closure of Skegness retreat complex.* [online]

https://www.derbytelegraph.co.uk/news/derby-news/miners-up-arms-over-closure-1934952

Granger, B. and Albu, S. 2011. *The Haloperidol Story.* [online]

    https://www.tandfonline.com/doi/abs/10.3109/10401230591002048

Jarlais, J. 2019. *Head banging: Why it happens and what to do about it.* [online]

    https://cutt.ly/0gPFdTA

Medical eStudy. 2018. *Common Psychotropic Drugs.* [online]

    http://www.medicalestudy.com/wp-content/uploads/2018/05/Psychotropic-Drugs.png

OMNIA. no date. *Headingley Castle.* [online]

    https://cutt.ly/OgPFbmN

Dry Slope News. no date. *Former Slopes.* [online]

    https://dryslopenews.com/former-slopes/

London OT. no date. *Activities of Daily Living Assessment.* [online]

    https://www.londonot.co.uk/services/assessment/activities-of-daily-living-assessment.php

Singing Hands. no date. *What is Makaton?* [online]

    https://singinghands.co.uk/about/what-is-makaton/

Drugs.com. 2020. *Baclofen.* [online]

    https://www.drugs.com/baclofen.html

Drugs.com. 2019. *Pregabalin.* [online]

    https://www.drugs.com/mtm/pregabalin.html

Drugs.com. 2020. *Carbamazepine.* [online]

    https://www.drugs.com/carbamazepine.html

Canehill. no date. *Cane Hill Hospital.* [online]

    https://cutt.ly/BgPGbw1